HEALTH CARE ISSUES, COSTS AND ACCESS

BIRTH DEFECTS: ISSUES ON PREVENTION

NEVIN HOTUN SAHIN
AND
ILKAY GUNGOR

Nova Science Publishers, Inc.
New York

NOTICE TO THE READER

The Publisher has taken reasonable care in the preparation of this book, but makes no expressed or implied warranty of any kind and assumes no responsibility for any errors or omissions. No liability is assumed for incidental or consequential damages in connection with or arising out of information contained in this book. The Publisher shall not be liable for any special, consequential, or exemplary damages resulting, in whole or in part, from the readers' use of, or reliance upon, this material.

Independent verification should be sought for any data, advice or recommendations contained in this book. In addition, no responsibility is assumed by the publisher for any injury and/or damage to persons or property arising from any methods, products, instructions, ideas or otherwise contained in this publication.

This publication is designed to provide accurate and authoritative information with regard to the subject matter covered herein. It is sold with the clear understanding that the Publisher is not engaged in rendering legal or any other professional services. If legal or any other expert assistance is required, the services of a competent person should be sought. FROM A DECLARATION OF PARTICIPANTS JOINTLY ADOPTED BY A COMMITTEE OF THE AMERICAN BAR ASSOCIATION AND A COMMITTEE OF PUBLISHERS.

Additional color graphics may be available in the e-book version of this book.

Library of Congress Cataloging-in-Publication Data
Sahin, Nevin Hotun.
  Birth defects issues on prevention / Nevin Hotun Sahin and Ilkay Gungor.
    p. ; cm.
  Includes bibliographical references and index.
  ISBN 978-1-61668-967-4 (softcover)
  1. Abnormalities, Human--Prevention. I. Gungor, Ilkay. II. Title.
  [DNLM: 1. Congenital Abnormalities--prevention & control. 2. Maternal
Health Services. 3. Socioeconomic Factors. QS 675 S131b 2010]
  RA645.A24S24 2010
  616'.043--dc22
                        2010025429

Published by Nova Science Publishers, Inc. ✝ *New York*

HEALTH CARE ISSUES, COSTS AND ACCESS

FEC TS:

VE TION

HEALTH CARE ISSUES, COSTS AND ACCESS

Additional books in this series can be found on Nova's website under the Series tab.

Additional E-books in this series can be found on Nova's website under the E-book tab.

Contents

Preface

Birth defects including genetic diseases contribute a significant proportion of infant morbidity and mortality and affect many parents and families. Every year 2–6% of newborns are born worldwide with major congenital anomalies and the majority of identified causes of congenital anomalies are nonhereditary and preventable. Theoretically, some of the risk to the developing fetus can be eliminated by avoiding exposure to the agent or manipulating the fetal environment. The main preventive measures recommended are expansion of rubella immunization, access to family planning programs that include the encouragement to complete reproduction before 35 years of age, periconceptional supplementation of folic acid, iodization of salt, and access to adequate prenatal care, including nutrition, control of maternal infections and avoidance of teratogens.

Ideally, prevention of fetal exposure to harmful influences begins before conception because all major organ systems develop early in pregnancy, often before a woman realizes that she is pregnant. During this period; health professionals can help make women aware of their need for a supplement of folic acid before conception to help reduce the risk of neural tube defects and teach a pregnant woman about harmful factors in her lifestyle that can be modified to reduce the risk of defects to offspring. Appropriate preconceptional and prenatal medical therapy can also help a woman prevent fetal damage that could result from her illness or medication such as diabetes, phenylketonuria, hypothyroidism, epilepsy etc. Social determinants of women's health also play a role in birth outcome. Low socioeconomic and educational level is related with increased incidence of malnutrition, mineral and vitamin deficiencies, and intrauterine infections, unsafe working conditions during gestation, and access to medicines without medical indication or prescription and common use of home remedies of unknown compositions. In addition, consanguineous marriages, which are known to increase the risk for birth defects, are acceptable and even common in many cultures.

As a consequence, it is essential to have basic information on the prevention of congenital anomalies and the roles of health professionals in order to provide effective counseling during the reproductive years. The purpose of this book is to present an overview of essential aspects of primary prevention efforts and effecting factors including age and socio-demographical factors, obstetric history, maternal medical conditions, genetic disorders, psycho-social issues, infections and vaccination, teratogenic agents, environmental risk factors, nutrition, folic acid supplementation, lifestyle factors, smoking, alcohol, maternal obesity, family planning, assisted reproduction techniques, culture and preconceptional care.

Introduction

More than 4 million children are born with birth defects each year. Although individually rare, birth defects taken together account for a significant proportion of morbidity and mortality among infants and children, particularly in areas where infant mortality due to more common causes has been reduced. The prevalence of specific conditions varies widely in different populations. In countries where basic public health services are not available, the birth prevalence of serious birth defects is generally higher than in developed countries. Today there is an unprecedented opportunity to prevent many birth defects and reduce the consequences of those that occur, and to do so at reasonable cost. A number of successful measures for the prevention of congenital anomalies are being taken in a number of developing nations. Primary prevention programs are based on public education about preconceptional and prenatal risks. The goal of primary prevention is to reduce the birth prevalence of congenital anomalies through the removal of causative factors. The majority of identified causes of congenital anomalies are nonhereditary, and the main preventive measures recommended include access to family planning programs that include the encouragement to complete reproduction before 35 years of age; access to adequate prenatal care, including nutrition, control of maternal infections and avoidance of teratogens; periconceptional supplementation of folic acid; expansion of rubella immunization; iodization of salt; appropriate counseling and screening in consanguineous marriages; avoidance of alcohol and smoking and promoting healthy lifestyle. Prenatal diagnosis and subsequent termination of affected pregnancies, as well as in-utero treatment of prenatally detected congenital anomalies, are two secondary preventive strategies. As the scope of in-utero treatment remains limited, secondary prevention is mainly achieved through selective abortion. Prenatal diagnosis also contributes to tertiary prevention in cases where an early prenatal diagnosis improves postnatal management and reduces or avoids neonatal complications. Effective strategies to address birth defects in developing countries must take into account the competing needs for resources and social, economic, and other factors that constrain health care resources. Health care systems and services vary widely both among and within countries. Thus to be effective, strategies and interventions need to be tailored to the specific population being served.

The purpose of this book is to present an overview of essential aspects of primary prevention efforts and effecting factors including age and socio-demographical factors, obstetric history, maternal medical conditions, genetic disorders, psycho-social issues, infections and vaccination, teratogenic agents, environmental risk factors, nutrition, folic acid supplementation, lifestyle factors, smoking, alcohol, maternal obesity, family planning, assisted reproduction techniques, culture and preconceptional care.

Chapter I

Demographical and Social Factors

Parental Age

There is an association between maternal age and the risk of chromosomal abnormalities [1,2] (Figure 1). The association between prevalence rates of birth defects and maternal age demonstrate a higher proportion of malformed children among women aged less than 20 years or more than 35 years. This is especially true for chromosomal abnormalities among women of advanced ages and disruptive malformation among teenage mothers [3]. Women over 35 years also experience an increased risk for several nonchromosomal defects, although not as high as their risk for chromosomal defects [4,5].

Croen and Shaw [6] found that the overall prevalence of all congenital anomalies across the age distribution was shown as a J shape, with women aged 20–29 years having the lowest prevalence, teenage women having an intermediate prevalence and women more than 40 years old having the highest prevalence. The prevalence of non-chromosomal anomalies tended to be a U-shaped curve, because the prevalence dropped substantially for women more than 40 years of age and only marginally for other age groups, after excluding chromosomal anomalies.

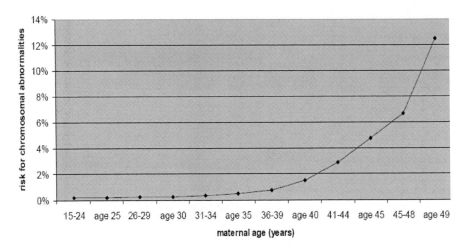

Figure 1. Maternal age and risk for any chromosomal abnormalities.

Advanced Maternal Age

The term "elderly parturient" was defined in 1958 by the Council of International Federations of Obstetrics as "one aged 35 years or more at the first delivery". Advanced maternal age has traditionally been defined as age > 35 years at delivery and a woman 45 years of age or older is considered to be of very advanced maternal age [7,8].

Over the past several decades, delayed childbirth has become a common phenomenon in the developed world as a result of economic, educational, technologic and social changes and the number of men and women who delay childbirth to their late 30s and beyond have significantly increased. A woman's career priorities, advanced education, infertility, control over fertility, late and second marriages, and financial concerns may play a role in delaying childbearing [7,9,10]. In a qualitative study involving women aged 20–48 years, independence, motivation to have a family, declining fertility, chronic health problems and stable relationships were identified as personal influences on decisions about the timing of child-bearing [11]. Pregnancies at advanced maternal ages are only partially the results of planned postponement of motherhood as a good percentage are secondary to infertility (20%) or to previous fetal losses (40%) [8].

Between 1980 and 1993 in the European Union, the mean maternal age at first birth rose by 1.5 years, from 27.1 to 28.6 years. Between 1991 and 2001 in the United States, the percentage of first births for women 35–39 years of age increased by 36% and that for women 40–44 years of age increased by 70% [10]. Live births in women >35 years of age increased from 5% in 1970 to 13% of all live births in 2000. Between 1977 and 1998, the number of women giving birth at 35 to 39, 40 to 44, and >45 years increased 9.9, 9.1, and 49.9 times, respectively. In 1999, the birth rate for women aged 40 to 44 years was the highest in almost two decades. Over 10 years, the average age at first delivery increased from 25.9 to 27.5 years and at any delivery from 27.3 to 29.7. This trend of postponing childbearing has not yet shown any tendency to decrease [8].

The frequency of birth defects is highest among mothers aged 35 years and over. These women have approximately a 20% increased risk of having a pregnancy affected by a birth defect compared to women less than 35 years of age. A women who is 40 years and over had almost a 60% increased risk of having a pregnancy affected by a birth defect compared to women less than 40 years of age. Tetralogy of Fallot, ventricular septal defect, cleft palate, cleft lip and palate, exomphalos, trisomy 21, trisomy 18 and trisomy 13 are all more likely to occur with older mothers [12]. Pregnancy at ≥35 and ≥40 years of age is thought to add 1% and 2.5% respectively to the risk of nonchromosomal malformations compared with the baseline risk of 3.5% in women <25 years of age. Those malformations include cardiac defects (2X), clubfoot (3X), and diaphragmatic hernia (10.5X), spina bifida, cleft palate, syndactyly, limb defects, and male genital malformation [8].

The simplest means of preventing Down syndrome and other chromosomal disorders such as trisomies 13 and 18 is to decrease the number of pregnancies among women older than 35 years. This is accomplished by making family planning widely available and providing information about risks. Access to family planning programs that include the encouragement to complete reproduction before 35 years of age should be improved and women should be discouraged from reproducing after age 35 to minimize the risk of chromosomal birth defects. This strategy was shown to be effective in Europe between 1950 and 1975 when family planning programs were expanded and the birth prevalence of Down syndrome decreased from 2.5 to 1.0 per 1,000 live births [13,14].

Young Maternal Age

Since the mid-1980s, pregnancy and birth rates among American teenagers have been increasing, with an estimated 11% of all women between the ages of 15 and 19 becoming pregnant, half of whom go on to deliver a live-born infant. This issue deserves attention, particularly given that low birth weight and infant mortality are outcomes for which infants of teen mothers are at high risk. Congenital malformations are associated with low birth weight and are the leading cause of infant mortality. Furthermore, factors suspected of playing a role in the etiology of some malformations such as poor diet, illicit drug use, and smoking may be more common during the pregnancies of young mothers than during those of older mothers [6].

As with older mothers, when considering the overall risk of structural birth defects, there is a significant association with increased odds of birth defects and maternal age less than 20 years of age. In mothers younger than 15 years old, the prevalence of these abnormalities is anywhere from 37 to 46.9 per 1000 births. This translates to an extra 27 birth defects per 1000 births when compared with mothers aged 25-29 years old who have the lowest risk [15].

In large database study it was demonstrated that the teenage pregnancy associated increase in risk for central nervous system anomalies was mainly attributable to anomalies other than anencephalus, spina bifida/meningocele and hydrocephalus and microcephalus; for gastrointestinal anomalies the risk was mainly attributable to omphalocele/gastroschisis; and for musculo-skeletal/integumental anomalies the risk was mainly attributable to cleft lip/palate and polydactyly/syndactyly/adactyly [16].

Although the etiology of some congenital anomalies needs further study, some lifestyle related factors associated with increased risk of congenital anomalies in teenage pregnancy offer us some opportunity for prevention. If teenage mothers get adequate prenatal care, have a healthy diet, avoid exposure to smoke, alcohol and drugs and take timely multivitamin and folic acid supplements, some of these congenital anomalies may be prevented [5].

Age-Related Factors

Maternal age, either young or advanced, is associated with several known risk factors for birth defects such as smoking, lack of prenatal care, inadequate health insurance, and the use of prenatal vitamins. There may be some biological reasons why young mothers are at a higher risk for birth defects, but lifestyle factors like smoking, alcohol, and illicit drug use seem to be the most likely explanation. Reported multivitamin use increases with increasing age among reproductive aged women and younger reproductive aged women have the lowest awareness of folic acid. In addition, young pregnant women have a lower intake of micronutrients. Subfertility and the use of fertility treatments have been associated with some types of defects and the prevalence of infertility increases with age. Maternal body mass also increases with age and pre-pregnancy obesity has been associated with certain birth defects. Finally, younger women are far more likely to have no health insurance coverage. This lack of health insurance may lead to inadequate or absent prenatal care [5]. The overall birth prevalence of chromosome disorders is higher in developing countries, resulting probably from the lack of family planning services and a higher proportion of births to women of advanced age. Indeed, the percentage of births to women over 35 years old ranges from 11 to 15% in different regions of the developing world, compared with 5–9% in industrialized countries. The very limited availability of, and access to, prenatal diagnosis and the fact that in many developing countries abortion is illegal further contribute to a higher birth prevalence of chromosome abnormalities [14].

Traditionally, screening and diagnostic tests for chromosomal abnormalities were offered to women over the age of 35, during the first or second or both trimesters of pregnancy. However, the age of 35 will no longer be the cutoff to determine when screening should be offered, because American College of Obstetricians & Gynecologists recently recommended offering all pregnant women genetic screening tests. This change is due to the variety of available screening tests with high detection rates and low false-positive rates and the good diagnostic options if the screening is positive [17].

Paternal Age

Although the association between maternal age and the risks of birth defects has been well studied, the role of paternal age has received relatively little attention. However, the risk of birth defects in general and several selected birth defects, such as heart malformation, other musculo skeletal/integumental anomalies, tracheo-oesophageal fistula/oesophageal atresia, Down's syndrome and other chromosomal anomalies, increases slightly with advancing paternal age. Accumulated chromosomal aberrations and mutations occurring during the maturation of male germ cells are thought to be responsible for the increased risk of certain conditions with older fathers. Growing evidence shows the offspring of older fathers have reduced fertility and an increased risk of birth defects, some cancers, and schizophrenia.

Association between younger fathers and several selected birth defects also exists [9,18].

The association of advanced paternal age with increased risk of mutations is less clear as the paternal contribution to fetal aneuploidy is not fully understood. It seems that the proportion of aneuploid cell in men is not a reliable indicator of the tendency to meiotic and somatic nondisjunction. It has been shown that during meiosis, 62% of nondisjunction events occur as a result of an error in the first maternal meiotic division, 15% in the second maternal meiotic division, 12% in the first paternal meiotic division, and 11% in the second paternal meiotic division. Most chromosomal unbalanced abortions are the result of maternal nondisjunction. All populations are at risk. The relative increased risk for these defects is related to advanced age of the father for autosomal dominant conditions and the maternal grandfather for X-linked conditions [19].

In a study, the incidence of chromosome aberrations was found higher when the age and birth order of parents are higher. A direct correlation was noted with parental order and the frequency of breaks per cell. This was also true with the parental age and birth defects. Children with chromosome anomalies were more frequent in parents with increased age and/or high parental birth order [19].

Ethnicity

The prevalence of specific birth defects varies widely with the ethnic, geographic, cultural, and economic characteristics of populations [13]. The inherited disorders for which carrier screening is currently recommended are Cystic fibrosis (Caucasian, Northern Europeans, Celtic population, Ashkenazi Jewish), Tay Sachs (Ashkenazi Jewish, Cajun, French Canadian), Canavan disease (Ashkenazi Jewish), Familial dysautonomia (Ashkenazi Jewish), Beta thalassemia (Mediterranean, Southeast Asian; Greek, Italian), Alpha thalassemia (Southeast Asian; Vietnamese, Loation, Cambodian, Filipino), Sickle cell anemia (African, African American; Hispanic from Caribbean, Central America, South America; Arabs, Egyptians, Asian Indians). There are many other disorders for which screening is available, including fragile X syndrome, as well as panels of diseases more common in the Ashkenazi Jewish population [20,21,22,23].

Carrier screening for specific genetic conditions often is determined by an individual's ancestry. Many populations are characterized by unusually high frequencies of particular single gene conditions. In some countries with high prevalence of hemoglobinopathies, there are population based prevention programs for the detection of carriers. Health education of the public, community involvement, carrier detection in general population, genetic counseling, testing of marrying couples and comprehensive prenatal diagnosis program are suggested strategies for prevention in the specific ethnic groups [24]. For example, carrier testing for serious autosomal recessive genetic disorders began in the early 1970s for Tay-Sachs disease (TSD), a lethal lysosomal storage disorder with a high carrier frequency (3%) in Ashkenazi Jewish individuals (Eastern European origin) and community-based screening programs have identified thousands of carrier couples who have been offered genetic counseling and a variety of reproductive options, including prenatal testing. As a result of this screening program, the incidence of TSD has dramatically declined, and this has served as a model for subsequent carrier screening programs [23].

According to the recommendations of ACOG Committee on Genetics [20]; individuals with a positive family history of one of these disorders should be offered carrier screening for the specific disorder and may benefit from genetic counseling. When both partners are carriers of one of these disorders, they should be referred for genetic counseling and offered prenatal diagnosis. Carrier couples should be informed of the disease manifestations, range of severity, and available treatment options. Prenatal diagnosis by DNA-based testing can be performed on cells obtained by chorionic villous sampling and amniocentesis. When an individual is found to be a carrier, his or her relatives are at risk for carrying the same mutation. The patient should be encouraged to inform his or her relatives of the risk and the availability of carrier screening [20].

Socioeconomic Status

Social position has been associated with a variety of health outcomes, related to perinatal and infant health, including congenital anomalies. An increased propensity to give birth to a child with a congenital anomaly has been reported for women with lower social position, as compared with better-off women. The association between social position and the risk of congenital anomalies is birth defect specific. Low social position is associated with increased risk of neural tube defects, orofacial clefts and transposition of the great arteries. On the other hand, there is a reduced risk of tetralogy of Fallot among the offspring of women with low social position [25]. Existing evidence suggests that most non-chromosomal anomalies increase in prevalence with increasing socioeconomic disadvantage [26].

Wealth or higher education in itself is unlikely to directly affect the occurrence of congenital anomalies, but low socioeconomic status may affect pregnancy outcome through a number of mechanisms. Unfavorable social conditions may influence health by forcing people into poor housing, heavy jobs or specific unhealthy environmental exposure. Low social position is a marker for unhealthy lifestyle, and the mother's social background and education may influence her compliance with public healthcare services and the use of healthcare facilities such as prenatal screening [14,25].

Many risk factors in the lower socioeconomic group of the population in developing countries can be prevented with good pre-conception and prenatal care [27]. Despite the existence of low-cost interventions for preventing and treating a number of birth defects, the human, economic, and social burdens associated with these conditions remain high. Obstacles to improving care for birth defects include financial constraints; lack of knowledge on the part of health care workers; poor access to medical facilities; and issues surrounding ethnicity, language, religion, and culture. Governments must be educated on the cost-effectiveness of reducing the impact of birth defects through proven methods of prevention and care, which can be adapted to local resources and needs [13].

The emphasis on individualized, holistic prenatal care, encompassing physiologic and psychosocial needs, promotes a prevention-oriented model of care. Today's families may face unemployment, homelessness, chemical dependency, increased family and neighborhood violence, and lack of support systems that may precipitate crises and affect perinatal outcome. Early recognition of potential risk allows for prompt intervention and referral. The role of the perinatal social worker is critical in providing interventions that relieve stress, providing for woman's basic needs, following crisis situations, and facilitating healthcare decision making [28].

Employment

Maternal employment potentially affects all stages of pregnancy, including possibly the incidence of congenital malformation. Known teratogens in the workplaces include lead, carbon monoxide and ionizing radiation. Also, health-care workers are considered particularly vulnerable to adverse pregnancy outcome where there is potential for exposure to biological hazards such as cytotoxic drugs, anaesthetic gases, mercury, ethylene oxide (used in the sterilization of hospital equipment) and ionizing radiation [29]. There have been reports of specific type of birth defects associated with certain maternal occupations. This observation also is true for certain paternal occupations. For example, maternal organic solvent exposure and paternal occupation of janitors and have been reported to be associated with ventricular septal closure defects. Mothers employed in a nursing occupation had excess risk of having urinary system defects. Paternal pesticide appliers were reported to have an elevate risk of musculoskeletal anomalies in offspring. Chromosomal anomalies other than Down's syndrome were reported to be associated with female medical radiographer and office machine operators. A notable and significant association between oral clefts and mothers involved in leather and shoe manufacturing was found. Fathers worked as painters were reported to have relationship with cleft palate [30]. In a review of epidemiological studies on paternal occupations and birth defects, there were several common paternal occupations that were repeatedly reported to be associated with birth defects. These paternal occupations were janitors, painters, printers, and occupations exposed to solvents; fire fighters or firemen; and occupations related to agriculture [31].

Maternal occupation should be evaluated for potential teratogenic exposures. Ministries of public health, in collaboration with other government departments in developing countries, should establish regulations to reduce occupational exposure to teratogens—such as mercury and other pollutants—and create programs to raise public awareness of the health risks, including birth defects, associated with these substances [13].

Abuse and Violence

Violence against women is an unfortunate fact of life for millions of women around the world. The lifetime physical or sexual intimate partner violence or both vary from 15% to 71% in many countries [32,33]. Pregnant women are at risk for physical violence inflicted by intimate partners. Although estimates in public and private health-care settings indicate that 4%-17% of women experience violence during pregnancy, population-based prevalence estimates of this problem have not been available. At least 4–8% of women report the violence during pregnancy [34]. Intimate partner violence is a common occurrence in pregnancy and results in an increased risk of adverse outcomes [35]. Violence during pregnancy may be more common than gestational diabetes, NTDs and preeclampsia. Frequently, the abuse begins during pregnancy, and battering is believed to cause more birth defects than all the conditions for which children now are immunized [36].

Women who are pregnant and the victims of violence have specific risk factors for birth defects including high rates of stress, high levels of anxiety and depression that often led to smoke, use alcohol or other drugs. Violence on pregnant women significantly increased risk for low birth weight infants, preterm delivery, infectious complications, unintended pregnancy, multiple abortions and neonatal death. Women battered by violence are less likely to obtain prenatal care. Adolescents may be at even higher risk than their adult counterparts [17,33,37].

Violence directed by an intimate partner toward the pregnant woman and her fetus, or during the first year after delivery, is often either not recognized by professionals or suspected but not addressed. There is no typical abused woman; in fact, intimate partner violence occurs across all social, economic, educational, and professional settings. Physical or sexual abuse may be readily observed in some instances or well hidden at other times; the emotional components of verbal, economic, and isolation abuse are often difficult to assess. All types of intimate partner violence require sensitive assessment and intervention by healthcare providers, as numerous undesirable outcomes for both the mother and her fetus/baby have been identified [37]. Healthcare providers, particularly those who care for pregnant women, are in a unique position to identify these women and direct them and their families to the help they need to end the violence in their lives [35].

Health caregiver needs to extend their interventions for the pregnant patient disclosing violence against women while treating their physical and emotional complaints to avoid adverse pregnancy outcomes. Women's efforts to seek safety from abuse may help to improve pregnancy outcomes and promote maternal welfare [33]. Healthcare providers may screen for violence against women related to possible demographic and psychosocial factors when evaluating the woman [38,39,40] (Table 1, Table 2). If a clinician chooses to screen for violence against women during routine woman in prenatal visits, a series of questions has been proposed as a means of evaluating the risk of violence against women [36]. Routine screening for violence against women remains controversial, in part because the benefit of screening, even with intervention, and the lack of any harm related to the screening have not been established definitively [36].

Table 1. Possible Factors and Effects of Violence

Possible Demographic/Psychosocial Factors	Routinely Screen Every Pregnant
<ul><li>Young maternal age/adolescence</li><li>Unintended pregnancy</li><li>Delayed prenatal care</li><li>Smoking</li><li>Alcohol and drug use</li><li>Lack of social supports</li><li>STD/HIV/AIDS</li></ul>	<ul><li>At least once per trimester</li><li>At postpartum checkup</li><li>At routine ob-gyn visits and preconception visits</li></ul>
Components of Screening	**Abuse Assessment Screen**
<ul><li>Review medical history.</li><li>Observe and record presentations and behaviors of pregnant and partner.</li><li>Ask direct questions and listen actively.</li><li>Document pregnant's response.</li></ul>	<ul><li>Explain issues of confidentiality</li><li>Short</li><li>Apart from male partner</li><li>Apart from family or friends</li><li>Tested in clinical settings</li><li>Effective in identifying violence</li></ul>Routinely ask every women;<ul><li>Ask directly, kindly, nonjudgmentally</li><li>**Report** your findings</li><li>Assess the pregnant's safety</li><li>Review options and provide referrals</li></ul>
Possible Effects on Fetus	
<ul><li>Direct effects<ul><li>spontaneous abortion</li><li>fetal injury or death from maternal trauma</li></ul></li><li>Indirect effects<ul><li>maternal stress</li><li>maternal smoking</li><li>alcohol / drug use or abuse</li></ul></li></ul>	

Efforts in preventing violence must be addressed at three separate, but connected, levels. These include three levels:

1. Primary prevention of violence by working within society;
2. Secondary prevention of continuing violence by assessing the women and providing information and decision-making guidance; and
3. Tertiary prevention of continuing abuse by providing women support and guidance for removing themselves (and any children) to a safe place [37]

The Joint Commission on Accreditation of Healthcare Organizations recommends that accredited emergency departments establish policies, procedures, and education programs to guide staff in the treatment of battered adults [41]. Furthermore, all healthcare providers should establish relations with organizations that can provide battered women with referral services such as acute care, legal aid, health care, and support groups.

Table 2. Sample Questions of Screen for Violence Against Women

Questions	
1.	Do you feel safe in your relationship?
2.	Are you afraid of your partner or anyone else?
3.	In the last year (since I saw you last), have you been hit, slapped, kicked, or otherwise physically hurt by someone? (If yes, by whom? Number of times? Nature of injury?)
4.	Since you've been pregnant, have you been hit, slapped, kicked, or otherwise physically hurt by someone? (If yes, by whom? Number of times? Nature of injury?)
5.	Within the last year has anyone made you do something sexual that you didn't want to do? (If yes, who?)
6.	Are you now or have you ever been in a relationship in which you have been physically hurt or threatened?
7.	What happens when you and your partner have a disagreement? How do you handle conflict? Does it ever get physical
8.	Has your partner ever prevented you from leaving the house, going out with friends, seeking employment, or continuing your education?
9.	Are you an equal partner when it comes to making important decisions that affect your family?

Culture and Traditions

Cultural beliefs and practices can affect the health status of the woman by influencing her use of healthcare services, confidence in and acceptance of recommended prevention and treatment strategies, and global beliefs regarding her body, illness, religion and so forth. Not every individual in a culture may display certain characteristics, as there are variations among cultures. Healthcare practices during pregnancy are influenced by numerous factors, such as consanguinity, viewing pregnancy as a natural occurrence, nutritional practices, beliefs about medications, use of home remedies and indigenous healers and seeking prenatal care [28].

In the developing world, the role of tradition in shaping health beliefs and patterns of health care is very strong. The structure of the family assigns as important authority role to the elders, and members of the extended family are active in decision making regarding health. The various cultural meanings of disease and causal explanations affect decisions regarding prevention and treatment. Although religion plays an important guiding role everywhere in the world, its directives tend to be more rigid, authoritarian and conservative in the developing countries than in the industrialized ones [24].

Consanguinity

A small proportion of congenital anomalies are due to single gene mutations, usually in the form of syndromes of multiple congenital anomalies. Although most of these conditions are rare, geographical clusters of unusually high frequencies of specific single gene congenital syndromes may occur due to demographic factors such as founder effects, genetic isolation or consanguinity. In some cases, these clusters can pose a significant public health concern [14]. In developing countries, the higher rate of traditional consanguineous marriages increases the frequency of autosomal recessive disorders with large family size, which may increase the number of affected children in families with autosomal recessive conditions [27]. Marriages between relatives are rare in industrially developed countries and also uncommon in Latin America and Eastern Asia; but they are highly prevalent in most Islamic countries, where, across a broad geographic area from Morocco to Pakistan, 20–80% of marriages are contracted between relatives. Not only Islam, but other religions also allow consanguineous marriages, to various degrees. The percentage of first cousin marriages among all marriages has been reported to be 11.4% in Egypt, 17% in Turkey, 30% in rural areas in the Islamic Republic of Iran, 29.2% in Iraq, 32% in Jordan, 30.2% in Kuwait, 17.3% among Muslim Lebanese and 7.9% among Christian Lebanese, 37.1% in Pakistan, 31.4% in Saudi Arabia and 30% in the United Arab Emirates [42,43]. Migrants from countries where consanguinity is common tend to preserve traditional patterns of marriage, especially if, in their new country, they remain disadvantaged by lower education or lower social class. Even in affluent groups, however, there may be social and economic advantages to marriage between relatives [43].

It is well known that offspring of consanguineous marriages are at increased risk for rare recessive syndromes, fetal, infant and child mortality, birth defects and later disabilities such as deafness, blindness, asthma, mental retardation or epilepsy. Consanguinity may also contribute to more distant outcomes, including some cancers in childhood and younger adults and complex diseases in later life [42,43]. The offspring of first cousin unions are estimated to have about a 1.7–2.8% increased risk for congenital defects above the population background risk. There is an approximately 4.4% increased risk for prereproductive mortality above the population background risk, some of which include major congenital defects. The risk for an adverse health outcome is greatest in the 1st year of life [44].

It is therefore often proposed that consanguineous marriage should be discouraged on medical grounds. However, several expert groups have pointed out that this proposal is inconsistent with the ethical principles of genetic counseling, overlooks the social importance of consanguineous marriage and is ineffective. Instead, they suggest that the custom increases the possibilities for effective genetic counseling, and recommend a concerted effort to identify families at increased risk, and to provide them with risk information and carrier testing when feasible [45,46].

A multicenter working group (the Consanguinity Working Group (CWG) with expertise in genetic counseling, medical genetics, biochemical genetics, genetic epidemiology, pediatrics, perinatology, and public health genetics, which was convened by the National Society of Genetic Counselors (NSGC) and the consensus of the CWG and NSGC reviewers is that beyond a thorough medical family history with follow-up of significant findings, no additional preconception screening is recommended for consanguineous couples. Consanguineous couples should be offered similar genetic screening as suggested for any couple of their ethnic group. During pregnancy, consanguineous couples should be offered maternal–fetal serum marker screening and high-resolution fetal ultrasonography. Newborns should be screened for impaired hearing and detection of treatable inborn errors of metabolism [44].

Remedies

Herbal remedies are therapeutic products and foods made from leaves, seeds, flowers and roots of plants or extracts of them. They are available in various forms, including teas, capsules, and tablets without prescription from a healthcare professional. Herbal remedies and alternative medicines are used throughout the world, and in the past herbs were often the original sources of most drugs. Today we are witnessing an increase in herbal remedy use throughout the western world raising the question as to how safe are these preparations for the unborn fetus? [47].

Many women use herbal products during pregnancy. Due to public perception, manufacturer contraindications, and recommendations by health care providers, pregnant women often avoid prescription and non-prescription drugs in pregnancy even when controlled trials cite safety. Many women use herbal products in pregnancy under the potentially false assumption that "natural" is synonymous with "safe." Inadvertent use may also occur because at least half of all pregnancies are not planned [48].

There are some herbs that are known teratogens that should under no circumstances be taken during pregnancy. Some herbs know to cause problems during pregnancy include, but are not limited to: Semen Crotonis (Ba Dou), Semen Pharbitidis (Qian Niu Zi), Radix Euphorbiae (Da Ji), Mulabris (Ban Mao), Radix Phytolaccae (Shang Lu), Moschus (She Xiang), Rhizoma Sparganii (San Leng), Rhizoma Zedoariae (EZhu), Hirudo seu Whitmania (Shui Zhi), and Tabanus (Meng Chong). Other herbs are recognized as potentially dangerous to the fetus and should be used with caution. Some of these include, but are not limited to Semen Persicae (Tao Ren), Flos Carthami (Hong Hua), Radix and Rhizomia Rhei (Da Huang) Fructus Aurantii (Zi Shi) Radix Aconiti (Fu Zhi), Rhizoma Zingiberis (Gan Jiang), and Cortex Cin namomi (Rou Gui) [47].

Some cultures in developing countries advocate home remedies of unknown composition and teratogenic potential, and in several developing countries, pharmaceutical companies market their products directly to consumers, who can purchase most medications over the counter without medical prescription [14]. Ensuring quality of herbal products should receive immediate attention by regulatory authorities, before embarking on the more arduous tasks of safety and efficacy [47].

Hyperthermia Associated with Hot Tub, Hammam, Sauna or SPA

Hot tub, SPA and sauna bathing are frequent among pregnant women in some countries. The Finnish-style sauna and the wet steam bath are the most widely known forms of sweat bathing. Many cultures have close equivalents, such as the North American First Nations sweat lodge, the Turkish hammam, Roman thermae, Aztec or Maya temazcal and Russian banya. In Finland and Russia sauna going plays a central social role. In Benelux and Scandinavian countries public saunas have been around for a long time too. During the past two decades, a series of retrospective and prospective epidemiological studies in humans has confirmed observations in experimental animals that suggested that hyperthermia could cause neural tube defects. The types of defects observed included spina bifida, encephalocele, and anencephaly. The sources of hyperthermia included febrile illnesses, sauna use, and hot tub use. Among these studies, the proportion of neural tube defects associated with first-trimester hyperthermia ranged from 10–14%. The relationship between exposure and neural tube defects was found stronger with hot tub use than with sauna use. Exposure to multiple heat sources was found to be associated with an even greater risk for neural tube defects [49,50,51].

A woman who knows or who may not yet be aware that she is pregnant should be advised of the recommended limits of exposure. She should also be aware of the possible variability in hot tub or SPA temperature readings and be able to accurately monitor maximum water temperature in the hot tub or spa so that her body temperature can be maintained below 38.98°C. [49,51]. For potentially pregnant women using hot tubs set at 40°C, exposure ought to be limited to no more than 10 min, while exposure in saunas set above 90°C ought to be limited to a maximum of 15 min. These limits appear to be commonly respected in countries such as Finland, where sauna-bathing is a way of life. Such countries demonstrate no excess of congenital defects that might be attributed to sauna-induced hyperthermia. It is only when these limits are not respected that the sauna might cause hyperthermia-induced defects [50].

References

[1]   ASRM- American Society for Reproductive Medicine. Age and Fertility. A Guide For Patients. 2003.

[2]   Metcalfe, SA; Barlow-Stewart, K; Delatycki, MB; Emery, J. Population genetic screening. *Aust. Fam. Physician.* 2007 Oct;36(10):794-800.

[3]   Nazer, HJ; Cifuentes, OL; Aguila, RA; Ureta, LP; Bello, PMP; Correa, CF; Melibosky, RF. The association between maternal age and congenital malformations. *Rev. Med. Chil.* 2007, 135(11), 1463-9.

[4]   Hollier, LM; Leveno, KJ; Kelly, MA; MCIntire, DD; Cunningham, FG. Maternal age and malformations in singleton births. *Obstet. Gyneco.* 2000, 96(5 Pt 1), 701-6.

[5]   Reefhuis, J; Honein, MA. Maternal age and non-chromosomal birth defects, Atlanta--1968-2000, teenager or thirty-something, who is at risk? *Birth Defects Res. A Clin. Mol. Teratol.* 2004, 70(9), 572-9.

[6]   Croen, LA; Shaw, GM. Young maternal age and congenital malformations: a population-based study. *Am. J. Public Health.* 1995 May;85(5):710-3.

[7]   Panchal, S. Considerations for the Parturient with Advanced Maternal Age: A Current Review the Society for Obstetric Anesthesia and

Perinatology, Available from: http://www.soap.org/media/newsletters/summer2001/current_review.ht m , Retrieved in 10.04.09

[8]   Usta, IM; Nassar, AH. Advanced maternal age. Part I: obstetric complications. *Am. J. Perinatol.* 2008, 25(8), 521-34.

[9]   Bray, I; Gunnell, D; Davey Smith, G. Advanced paternal age: how old is too old? *J. Epidemiol. Community Health.* 2006, 60(10), 851-3.

[10]   Huang, L; Sauve, R; Birkett, N; Fergusson, D; van Walraven, C. Maternal age and risk of stillbirth: a systematic review. *CMAJ.* 2008, 178(2), 165-72.

[11]   Benzies, KM. Advanced maternal age: are decisions about the timing of child-bearing a failure to understand the risks? *CMAJ.* 2008, 178(2), 183-4.

[12]   Halliday, J; Riley, M. Victorian Birth Defects Register Report − 2005. Victorian Birth Defects Bulletin. No. 3 June 2007.

[13]   Bale, JR; Stoll, BJ; Lucas, AO. Reducing Birth Defects: Meeting the Challenge in the Developing World. Washington, DC, National Academies Press, 2003.

[14]   Penchaszadeh, VB. Preventing Congenital Anomalies in Developing Countries. *Community Genet.* 2002, 5, 61–69.

[15]   Birth defects higher in older and younger women. http://www.ivf1.com 2009

[16]   Chen, XK; Wen, SW; Fleming, N; Yang, Q; Walker, MC. Teenage pregnancy and congenital anomalies: which system is vulnerable? *Hum. Reprod.* 2007 Jun;22(6):1730-5. Epub 2007 Mar 19.

[17]   ACOG-American College of Obstetricians and Gynecologists. New recommendations for Down syndrome call for screening of all pregnant women. Washington, DC, 2007.

[18]   Yang, Q; Wen, SW; Leader, A; Chen, XK; Lipson, J; Walker, M. Paternal age and birth defects: how strong is the association? *Hum. Reprod.* 2007, 22(3), 696-701.

[19]   Dinesh, RD; Pavithran, K; Henry, PY; Elizabeth, KE; Sindhu, P; Vijayakumar, T. Correlation of age and birth order of parents with chromosomal anomalies in children. *Genetika.* 2003 Jun;39(6):834-9.

[20]   ACOG- American College of Obstetricians and Gynecologists Committee Opinion No. 442: Preconception and prenatal carrier screening for genetic diseases in individuals of Eastern European Jewish descent. ACOG Committee on Genetics. *Obstet Gynecol.* 2009 Oct;114(4):950-3.

[21] Davidson, MR; London, ML; Ladewig, PW. Old's Maternal Newborn Nursing Women's Health Across the Lifespan. *Pearson-Prentice Hall.* New Jersey. 2008. p: 288-291.

[22] Norton, ME. Genetic screening and counseling. *Current Opinion in Obstetrics and Gynecology.* 2008, 20, 157–163.

[23] Vallance, H; Ford, J. Carrier testing for autosomal-recessive disorders. *Crit. Rev. Clin. Lab. Sci.* 2003 Aug;40(4):473-97.

[24] WHO: Prevention and care of genetic diseases and birth defects in developing countries (WHO/HGN/GL/WAOPBD/99.1). Geneva, WHO, 1999.

[25] Olesen, C; Thrane, N; Ronholt, AM; Olsen, J; Henriksen, TB. Association between social position and congenital anomalies: A population-based study among 19,874 Danish women. *Scand. J. Public Health.* 2009, doi:10.1177/1403494808100938.

[26] Dolk, H. Epidemiological Evidence Regarding Environmental Causes of Congenital Anomalies: Interpretational Issues. In: In: EUROCAT Special Report. The environmental causes of congenital anomalies: a review of the literature. [online]

[27] Rehman, A; Fatima, S; Soomro, N. Frequency of congenital anomalies and associated maternal risk factors in the lower socio-economic group. *Pakistan Journal of Surgery.* 2006, 22(3), 169-173.

[28] Simpson, KR; Creehan, PA. AWHONN's Perinatal Nursing: Co-Published with AWHONN (Simpson, Awhonn's Perinatal Nursing), 2008.

[29] Walker, SP; Higgins, JR; Permezel, M; Brennecke, SP; Phil, D. Maternal work and pregnancy. *Aust. N. Z. J. Obstet. Gynaecol.* 1999, 39(2), 144-51.

[30] Chia, SE; Shi, LM; Chan, OY; Chew, SK; Foong, BH. A population-based study on the association between parental occupations and some common birth defects in singapore (1994-1998). *J. Occup. Environ. Med.* 2004, 46(9), 916-23.

[31] Chia, SE; Shi, LM. Review of recent epidemiological studies on paternal occupations and birth defects. *Occup. Environ. Med.* 2002, 59(3), 149-55.

[32] Kendall-Tackett, KA. Violence Against Women and the Perinatal Period: The Impact of Lifetime Violence and Abuse on Pregnancy, Postpartum, and Breastfeeding. Trauma Violence Abuse, 2007, 8; 344.

[33] Sarkar, NN. The impact of intimate partner violence on women's reproductive health and pregnancy outcome. *Journal of Obstetrics and Gynaecology.* 2008, 28, 3,266-271.

[34] Mortaliy and morbiditiy Weekly Report.CDC. March 04, 1994 / 43(08);132-137.

[35] Chambliss, LR. Intimate partner violence and its implication for pregnancy. *Clin. Obstet. Gynecol.* 2008, 51(2), 385-97.

[36] Berkowitz, CD. Domestic Violence: A Pediatric Concern. *Pediatr. Rev.* 2004, 25, 306-311.

[37] Shoffner, DH. We Don't Like to Think About It Intimate Partner Violence During Pregnancy and Postpartum. *J. Perinat. Neonat. Nurs.* 2008, 22(1), 39–48.

[38] ACOG- American College of Obstetricians and Gynecologists and the U.S. Centers for Disease Control. Intimate Partner Violence During Pregnancy. A Guide for Clinicians.

[39] ACOG- American College of Obstetricians and Gynecologists.

[40] Melvin SY. Confronting the complex diagnosis of domestic violence. *Primary Care Rep.* 1995;1(3):21–28.

[41] Joint Commission on Accreditation of Healthcare Organizations. Accreditation manual for hospitals. Vol 1- standards. Oakbrook Terrace, Illinois: Joint Commission on Accreditation of Healthcare Organizations, 1992:21-2.

[42] Hamamy, H; Alwan, A. Genetic disorders and congenital abnormalities: strategies for reducing the burden in the Region. *Eastern Mediterranean Health Journal.* 1997, 3(1), 123-132.

[43] Harlap, S; Kleinhaus, K; Perin, MC; Calderon-Margalit, R; Paltiel, O; Deutsch, L; Manor, O; Tiram, E; Yanetz, R; Friedlander, Y. Consanguinity and birth defects in the jerusalem perinatal study cohort. *Hum. Hered.* 2008, 66(3), 180-9.

[44] Bennett, RL; Motulsky, AG; Huddgins, L; et al. Genetic counseling and screening of consanguineous couples and their offspring: Recommendations of the National Society of Genetic Counselors. *J. Genet. Couns.* 2002, 11(2):97–119.

[45] Modell, B; Darr, A. Science and society: genetic counselling and customary consanguineous marriage. *Nat. Rev. Genet.* 2002, 3(3), 225-9.

[46] Søgaard, M; Vedsted-Jakobsen, A. Consanguinity and congenital abnormalities] *Ugeskr. Laeger.* 2003, 165(18), 1851-5.

[47]   Rousseaux, CG; Schachter, H. Regulatory issues concerning the safety,
        efficacy and quality of herbal remedies. *Birth Defects Res. B. Dev.
        Reprod. Toxicol.* 2003, 68(6), 505-10.

[48]   Gallo, M; Einarson, A; Koren, G. Herbal medicine use in pregnancy: a
        new frontier in clinical teratology. *Birth Defects Res. B. Dev. Reprod.
        Toxicol.* 2003, 68(6), 499-500.

[49]   Chambers, CD. Risks of hyperthermia associated with hot tub or spa
        use by pregnant women. *Birth Defects Res. A Clin. Mol. Teratol.* 2006,
        76(8), 569-73.

[50]   Graham, JM; Jr Edwards, MJ; Edwards, MJ. Teratogen update:
        gestational effects of maternal hyperthermia due to febrile illnesses and
        resultant patterns of defects in humans. *Teratology.* 1998, 58(5), 209-
        21.

[51]   Moretti, ME, Bar-Oz, B; Fried, S; Koren, G. Maternal hyperthermia
        and the risk for neural tube defects in offspring: systematic review and
        meta-analysis. *Epidemiology.* 2005, 16(2), 216-9.

Chapter II

Genetic History
and Obstetric Factors

History of Genetic Conditions
and Risk of Recurrence

One way that heterogeneity of risk is expressed is as an increased recurrence among those who have already had the disease. For example, a couple whose first baby had a birth defect has about two to seven times the risk for the same defect in their next child compared with couples whose first baby had no defect. The first birth defect obviously does not cause the second; the higher risk at the second pregnancy reflects the presence of shared causes acting on both the first and second pregnancies. Having one baby with a birth defect does not necessarily mean a given couple is at higher risk in the next pregnancy – transient factors presumably play a role also. However, these couples clearly have a higher risk as a group [1].

Aneuploidies like Trisomy 21 (Down syndrome) generally have low recurrence risk. Women of advanced maternal age (> 35) are at increased risk for aneuploidy, regardless of family history. Chromosome translocations have variable recurrence risk, dependent on the specific chromosome material involved and whether translocation is familial or de novo. Autosomal recessive conditions have 25% recurrence risk in each subsequent pregnancy. Autosomal dominant conditions have 50% recurrence risk if inherited mutation, and low recurrence risk if de novo mutation. For X-linked conditions, if inherited mutation, male fetuses are at 50% risk of being affected and female fetuses have 50% risk of being a carrier; if de novo they have low recurrence risk. Multifactorial conditions (e.g., neural tube defects, cleft lip/palate, and congenital heart disease) have greater risk than general population and the risk is affected by many variables [2].

Unlike single gene traits, multifactorial disorders are not associated with fixed risk of occurrence or recurrence in a family. The risks are an average rather than a constant percentage. However, if no genetic component exists (if the disorder were totally related to environment), the ability to predict the risk for recurrence would be minimal. Factors that may affect the risk of recurrence; [3,4].

- *Number of affected close relatives:* Risk increases as the number of affected close relatives (parents, full sibling or child)
- *Severity of the disorder in affected family members:* For example, bilateral cleft lip is associated with a higher risk for recurrence in a close relative than is a unilateral cleft lip)
- *Sex of the affected persons:* For example, pyloric stenosis occurs five times as often in males as in females. The couple who has a doughter with pyloric stenosis faces a higher risk for recurrence with future children because the genetic influence for development of the defect is greater if a female develops it.
- *Geographic location:* The risk for some disorders such as neural tube defects is higher in some locations than others.
- *Seasonal variations:* Seasonal variations are noted with some multifactorial disorders.

Population-based studies indicated a greatly elevated risk of malformation recurrence among siblings of previously affected infants. Approximately two-fold increased risk are observed for the occurrence of any defect among women whose prior infant was malformed [5,6,7]. It is reported that among women whose first infant has a birth defect, the risk of the same defect in the second infant is substantially increases and the risk of a different defect in the second infant is slightly increases and also environment plays a strong part in repeated defects [6]. In a population-based study conducted using maternally linked birth certificate records from Washington, Mueller and Schwartz [7] found that women with a malformed infant had an increased risk of having a malformed infant at the subsequent birth, which did not vary by intervening changes in partner or residence. The risk of recurrence of the same general type of defect was much greater than that of occurrence of a dissimilar defect.

According to two population-based cohort studies of data from the Medical Birth Registry of Norway, women and girls with birth defects have decreased survival as compared with those with no birth defects, especially in the first years of life, and are less likely to have children. In addition, they have an increased risk of having children with the same defect. Compared with unaffected males, males with birth defects have higher mortality and survivors are less likely to have a child. Fathers with birth defects are significantly more likely than unaffected fathers to have an affected child [8,9].

Dependant on previous history, there is a relatively great diversity in the risk of recurrence. The prognosis of such disorders is very poor, therefore, their early recognition, and moreover, their prevention presents a key task for genetic counseling [10]. Preconceptional health promotion and intercom-ceptional counseling may be even more beneficial for parents who have had previous perinatal losses to evaluate genetic risks [2]. Counseling a couple after perinatal losses would be deficient without addressing the couple's future reproductive risks. To evaluate these risks, one must evaluate any medical, psychological, genetic, environmental, and obstetric concerns. It is important to discuss the chances of each possible outcome, including a recurrent loss and a normal birth, to help the parents put these risks into perspective [2].

History of Recurrent Miscarriages

It is well known that a negative selection exists against chromosomally abnormal offspring in nature. As a result of early preselection and subsequent pregnancy losses, the incidence of chromosomal abnormalities decreases with the advancing gestational age and successful pregnancy occurs in such a manner that the incidence of chromosomal abnormalities in live births is 0.6%,1 whereas the incidence in spontaneous abortions is around 50–70%. [11,12,13].

Recurrent spontaneous miscarriages affects up to one percent of the population, with approximately 90% presenting as missed abortions in the first trimester. Chromosomal aberrations such as aneuploidy account for approximately 50% of sporadic fetal losses prior to 15 weeks [14]. The major chromosomal abnormalities observed in spontaneous abortions are mostly numerical abnormalities, making up almost 95% of all anomalies. The most commonly detected numerical abnormalities in early pregnancy losses are autosomal trisomies, monosomy X and polyploidies. Among the trisomies, the most common ones occur in chromosomes 16, 22 and chromosome. Recurrent miscarriage is associated with a higher incidence of chromosomally abnormal embryos [11,12,13].

The impact of chromosomal abnormalities is greatest during fetal life when they have their highest frequency and represent a major cause of fetal loss. Chromosome abnormalities are present at least in 10% of all spermatozoa and 25% of mature oocytes. Approximately 50% of all spontaneous pregnancy loss and the loss of a very high proportion of all human conceptions are due to chromosome abnormalities. Genetic factors contribute to at least 40% of all congenital abnormalities with the major contribution being made by malformations showing multifactorial inheritance [14].

Parity

Investigators from several studies have reported a positive association between parity and Down's syndrome, although several other groups did not find an association [15,16,17]. The interpretation of many of these studies has been hindered by certain methodological issues. Because parity is closely correlated with maternal age, and because several early studies examining the relation between parity and Down's syndrome used broad (5-year) categories in controlling for maternal age, it has been suggested that at least part of the apparent effect of parity is due to residual confounding. Additionally, there is some evidence that women of higher parity are less likely to undergo prenatal screening for Down's syndrome by amniocentesis or chorionic villous sampling and therefore are less likely to choose to terminate a Down's syndrome pregnancy than women of lower parity. This would result in an excess of Down's syndrome livebirths among multiparous women, even in the absence of a true biologic association with parity [15,16]. However, in a case-control study, the authors used exact matching on maternal age–minimize confounding and evaluated the potential impact of differential termination. A total of 898 cases of Down's syndrome and 4,488 controls were identified using Washington State birth certificates from 1984–1998. There was a trend towards increasing risk of Down's syndrome with increasing parity in both younger (age <35 years) and older (age ≥35 years) mothers. Restriction to women with no indication of amniocentesis (for whom differential termination is unlikely) resulted in a blunting of the odds ratios; however, a trend for parity remained. Although the odds ratios for older women were probably biased upwards because of underreporting of amniocentesis on birth certificates, these data support an association between parity and Down's syndrome [16].

Complicated Situations
Related to Current Pregnancy

Preterm Birth

The relationship between birth defects and preterm birth is complex. Birth defects are associated with an increased risk of preterm birth, and babies born preterm have a higher likelihood of having a birth defect. Medical complications for infants born with birth defects can be compounded by prematurity because they are at greater risk for adverse events. In addition, some complications of preterm birth that develop after birth have long-term health consequences in childhood and adulthood that are similar to those among people with birth defects. As one example, there are a variety of etiologies for hearing loss, including genetic variants, environmental factors, and gene-environment interactions [18].

In a recent study from 13 states with population-based birth defects surveillance systems showed that birth defects were more than twice as common among preterm births (24–36 weeks) compared with term births (37–41 weeks gestation) and approximately 8% of preterm births had a birth defect. Birth defects were over five times more likely among very preterm births (24–31 weeks gestation) compared with term births, with about 16% of very preterm births having a birth defect. Defects most strongly associated with very preterm birth included central nervous system defects and cardiovascular defects [19].

The evidence presented thus far regarding birth defects and preterm birth suggests that in many cases an infant is at risk for not one but both outcomes simultaneously. Furthermore, some preventive measures and efforts to reduce risk factors can be expected to prevent both birth defects and preterm birth [18].

According to the March of Dimes and American College of Obstetricians and Gynecologists, here are some steps all women and health care providers can take before and during pregnancy to reduce the risk of birth defects and preterm birth, and to increase the chance of a healthy baby [20,21]:

1. Plan for pregnancy during a preconception visit that initiates the reduction of risk factors such as smoking and promotes healthy behaviors such as taking folic acid

2. Screen for and control medical conditions such as infection, diabetes, and high blood pressure
3. Review medications (prescription, over-the-counter, or home remedies) and modify as needed
4. Take a multivitamin with at least 400 micrograms of folic acid daily beginning before conception and continuing throughout pregnancy
5. Measure weight and height to calculate body mass index (BMI) before pregnancy. Discuss the need to be at a healthy weight before pregnancy and outline the ideal weight gain during pregnancy
6. Eliminate cigarette, alcohol, and illegal drug use
7. Take and review family history for any adverse birth outcomes, such as birth defects and preterm birth, and consider how it affects risk. Refer to a genetic counselor, if needed.

Multiple Pregnancies

Congenital anomalies are more common in twins than singletons but in the majority, etiology is not known. In a high quality, population-based study on multiple pregnancies and congenital anomalies found that twins, particularly monochorionic twins, have a higher risk of congenital anomalies than singletons [22]. A recent study tested the hypothesis that survivors of an early loss in a multiple conception, compared with all singletons, are at increased risk of congenital anomaly and found a highly significant increase in the risk of congenital anomaly in survivors from a multiple conception following early loss of a conceptus [23].

Obstetricians and parents should be aware of these risks associated with the obstetric history of women including parity, previous miscarriages and multiple pregnancies. In case of a high risk, parental karyotyping, in vitro fertilization plus pregestational diagnosis may be important steps in the management of these couples [11,12,13].

Amniotic Fluid Abnormalities

Changes in the amniotic fluid are strongly associated with congenital anomalies. Abnormal swallowing (obstruction or neurologic) means many fetuses with anomalies, including aneuploidy, have polyhydramnios. Abnormalities causing gastrointestinal obstruction, including tracheoesophageal (TE) fistula and esophageal atresia, may generate polyhydramnios of severe proportion for which antenatal imaging is often inconclusive. Others have underlying neurologic disorders and polyhydramnios due to absent or reduced swallowing. This is often associated with reduced activity, symmetric IUGR, and nongastrointestinal anomalies (e.g. cardiac anomalies, spina bifida, akinesia). Urinary tract anomalies such as urinary tract obstruction, renal failure, oliguria, placental failure, renal agenesis and absent lung fluid (tracheal atresia) are often related to decreased production of amniotic fluid and oligohydramnios. Interaction of multiple effects (for example, the fetus who has both a tracheoesophageal fistula and a renal dysplasia—reduced elimination and reduced production) may yield normal amniotic fluid volume in anomalous fetuses [24,25].

Intrauterine Growth Restriction (IUGR)

There is strong association between IUGR, chromosome aberrations and congenital malformations. Fetuses with chromosome disorders are frequently growth restricted, and suboptimal growth is also reported for many autosomal abnormalities such as duplications, deletions and ring chromosomes. It is thought that an abnormal fetal karyotype is responsible for approximately 20% of all IUGR fetuses, and the percentage is substantially higher if growth failure is detected before 26 weeks' gestation. It is likely that the compromised karyotype impairs normal cell division leading to a reduction in cell number and fetal growth [26].

Chromosomal abnormalities, such as trisomy 21 (Down syndrome), trisomy 18 (Edwards syndrome), trisomy 13 (Patau syndrome), and many others, can cause growth restriction presumably through the reduced number of small muscular arteries in the tertiary stem villi. IUGR can be as a result of or a reaction to the presence of malformations or it predisposes the fetus to malformations or else coexists with malformations because of common etiologic factors [27].

Macrosomia

Overgrowth syndromes are characterized by macrosomia, congenital anomalies, mental retardation and an increased risk of tumors. Several chromosomal abnormalities are associated with fetal overgrowth, including trisomy 12p, mosaic tetrasomy 12p (also known as Pallister-Killian syndrome), trisomy 4p16.3, trisomy 5p, trisomy 15q25, mosaic trisomy 8 and monosomy 22q13 [28].

In a case-control study comparing the birth weights of 8,226 infants with congenital anomalies ascertained by the Texas Birth Defects Monitoring Division with those of 965,965 infants without birth defects, infants with congenital anomalies were more likely than infants without birth defects to have a birth weight ≥4,500 g. Infants born with ventricular septal defects, atrial septal defects, ventricular hypertrophy, or anomalies of the great vessels were 1.5-2.5 times more likely to weigh ≥4,000 g than were infants without birth defects. Based on small numbers, a stronger excess of macrosomia was observed for infants with encephalocele, holoprosencephaly, anomalies of the corpus callosum, preaxial polydactyly, and omphalocele [29].

Detection of the large for gestational age fetus should first prompt the provider to rule out incorrect dates and maternal diabetes. Once this is done, consideration should be given to certain overgrowth syndromes, especially if anomalies are present. The overgrowth syndromes have significant clinical and molecular overlap, and are associated with developmental delay, tumors, and other anomalies [28].

Hyperbilirubinemia Related to Rh Isoimmunization, ABO Incompatibility and Prematurity

Hyperbilirubinemia may lead to the development of free bilirubin, that form of bilirubin which may cross the blood-brain barrier and enter and damage the basal nuclei of the brain. This rare, though devastating complication, may result in irreversible bilirubin induced brain damage termed kernicterus. Most cases of kernicterus are preventable. ABO blood group incompatibility is nowadays the most frequent cause of neonatal immune hemolytic disease. Kernicterus was a not uncommon occurrence prior to the 1970s, at which time the most frequent etiologic factor was Rh isoimmunization. Modern therapeutic techniques including exchange transfusion, phototherapy, the use of intravenous immune globulin therapy and maternal anti-D antibody (Rhogam) administration were instrumental in almost eliminating this condition [30].

Prevention of bilirubin encephalopathy is based on the detection of infants at risk of developing a significant hyperbilirubinemia. This task can be accomplished by performing a simple umbilical cord blood test, such as blood group, Rh, Coombs' test and glucose-6-phosphate dehydrogenase, in order to detect hemolytic diseases. In preterm infants, the prevention of hyperbilirubinemia with phototherapy is a relatively simple task, since these infants are cared for in hospital. Early hospital discharge of full-term neonates represents a major concern. The management of neonatal jaundice requires that therapy begins when total serum bilirubin levels are significantly below the levels at which kernicterus is considered an immediate threat. Full-term neonates who lose a significant amount of weight are especially at risk of significant hyperbilirubinemia and must be treated with ad libitum feeding and intensive phototherapy [31].

The American Academy of Pediatrics emphasizes paying attention to risk factors, including borderline prematurity, breast-feeding, and jaundice manifesting within the first 24 post-natal hours, and has recommended follow-up within 2 to 3 days of discharge to all neonates discharged before 48 h, and those born before 38 weeks of gestation [32].

Placental Abnormalities

Some investigators suggested an association between placental abnormalities and congenital anomalies and demonstrated that, pregnancies complicated with placenta previa and preterm placental abruption have significantly higher rates of congenital malformations [33,34]. For example, results of a population-based retrospective cohort study confirmed the association between placenta previa and congenital anomalies even after controlling for maternal age and other potential confounders. This finding might be important when assessing and counseling patients with placenta previa; however, the mechanism of the association is not known [33].

Preeclampsia

Since it has been demonstrated that reduced perfusion of the trophoblast, which is an early feature of preeclampsia, can also represent a cause of fetal malformation, there may be a positive correlation between the two conditions. In a retrospective examination of 8,894 cases, a higher incidence of preeclampsia was found in the presence of malformation. In addition, multivariate analysis showed that malformations of the male genital apparatus and those named 'multiple congenital abnormalities' can be considered as risk factors for preeclampsia. Since it is known that the development of male genitalia occurs under the influence of androgens, it can be hypothesized that hypoxia could act by favoring low end organ responsiveness [35].

Birth Trauma

The most frequently occurring newborn birth injuries include, hyphema, retinal hemorrhage, intracranial hemorrhage, fractured clavicle, cerebellar contusion, abducens nerve injury (cranial VI), skull fracture, phrenic nerve injury (3rd, 4th, and 5th cervical nerves), brachial plexus injuries, fractured femur, fractured humerus, facial palsy (cranial nerve VII), nasal septum deviation, laryngeal nerve injury, ruptured liver, subdural hematoma, subluxation of cervical spine, subgaleal hemorrhage, epiphysis separation and spinal cord injury [36].

Nearly half of major birth injuries and serious negative outcomes are potentially avoidable with early detection and intervention. The ability to decrease birth injuries partly reflects the technologic advancements that allow obstetricians and midwives to recognize perinatal risk factors for birth injury before attempting a vaginal delivery [36].

Some examples of perinatal risk factors that have been linked with birth injuries include large-for-date fetuses, especially fetuses who weigh more than 4500 g, deliveries requiring forceps or vacuum extractors, vaginal breech delivery, and deliveries that require abnormal or excessive traction during the birthing process. Factors responsible for mechanical injury can coexist with hypoxic-ischemic insults, with one predisposing the fetus to the other. Separating the effects of a fetus' hypoxic-ischemic insult from those of a traumatic birth injury is difficult and frequently impossible. Fetal anomalies are one of the important factors documented to predispose a fetus to birth injury. It is suggested that obstetricians should alert the pediatricians when these predisposing factors exist to aid in the recognition and early treatment of the birth injuries [36,37].

Intrapartum Asphyxia

When intrapartum asphyxia occurs, outcome can be very different depending on the duration and the extent of the asphyxia. Approximately 10–20% of children end up with a clinical picture of cerebral palsy. Many of these children develop cognitive and visual disturbances. Although the impact of intrapartum asphyxia seems to be relatively small compared with the effect of antenatal insults, major sequelae do occur after birth problems [38]. Neonatal complications of intrapartum asphyxia include multiorgan failure and neonatal encephalopathy. Most severe consequences are death and neurological or sensorial impairment [39].

Chorioamnionitis

Current evidence show that chorioamnionitis gives rise to a fetal inflammatory response, and that this inflammation contributes to neonatal brain injury and subsequent cerebral palsy. For example in a meta-analysis evaluating the relationship between chorioamnionitis and cerebral palsy, it was found that chorioamnionitis is a risk factor for both cerebral palsy and cystic periventricular leukomalacia [40].

References

[1]   Wilcox, AJ. The analysis of recurrence risk as an epidemiological tool. *Paediatr. Perinat. Epidemiol.* 2007, 21 Suppl 1, 4-7.

[2]   Wallerstedt, C; Lilley, M; Baldwin, K. Interconceptional counseling after perinatal and infant loss. *J. Obstet. Gynecol. Neonatal Nurs.* 2003, 32(4), 533-42.

[3]   Murray, SS; McKinney, ES. Foundations of Maternal Newborn Nursing. Fourth Edition, Saunders Elsevier, USA, 2006.

[4]   McKinney, ES; James, SR; Murray, SS; Ashwill, JW. *Maternal Child Nursing.* Saunders; Second edition, 2005.

[5]   Knox, EG; Lancashire, RJ. Epidemiology of Congenital Malformations. London: Her Majesty's Stationery Office, 1991.

[6]   Lie, RT; Wilcox, AJ; Skjaerven, R. A population-based study of the risk of recurrence of birth defects. *N. Engl. J. Med.* 1994, 7;331(1), 1-4.

[7]   Mueller, BA; Schwartz, SM. Risk of recurrence of birth defects in Washington State. *Paediatr. Perinat. Epidemiol.* 1997, 11 Suppl 1:107-18.

[8]   Lie, RT; Wilcox, AJ; Skjaerven, R. Survival and reproduction among males with birth defects and risk of recurrence in their children. *JAMA.* 2001, 285(6), 755-60.

[9]   Skjaerven, R; Wilcox, AJ; Lie, RT. A population-based study of
        survival and childbearing among female subjects with birth defects and
        the risk of recurrence in their children. *N. Engl. J. Med.* 1999, 340(14),
        1057-62.
[10]   Joó, JG; Beke, A; Papp, Z; Csaba, A; Rab, A; Papp, C. Risk of
        recurrence in major central nervous system malformations between
        1976 and 2005. *Prenat. Diagn.* 2007, 27(11), 1028-32.
[11]   Carp, HJ. Recurrent miscarriage: genetic factors and assessment of the
        embryo. *Isr. Med. Assoc. J.* 2008, 10(3), 229-31.
[12]   Christiansen, OB; Steffensen, R; Nielsen, HS; Varming, K.
        Multifactorial etiology of recurrent miscarriage and its scientific and
        clinical implications. *Gynecol. Obstet. Invest.* 2008, 66(4), 257-67.
[13]   Rubio, C; Pehlivan, T; Rodrigo, L; Simón, C; Remohí, J; Pellicer, A.
        Embryo aneuploidy screening for unexplained recurrent miscarriage: a
        minireview. *Am. J. Reprod. Immunol.* 2005, 53(4), 159-65.
[14]   Dinesh, RD; Pavithran, K; Henry, PY; Elizabeth, KE; Sindhu, P;
        Vijayakumar, T. Correlation of age and birth order of parents with
        chromosomal anomalies in children. *Genetika.* 2003 Jun;39(6):834-9.
[15]   Chan, A; McCaul, KA; Keane, RJ; Haan EA. Effect of parity,
        gravidity, previous miscarriage, and age on risk of Down's syndrome:
        population based study. *BMJ.* 1998, 317, 923–4.
[16]   Doria-Rose, VP; Kim, HS ; Augustine, ET; Edwards, KL. Parity and
        the risk of Down's syndrome. *Am. J. Epidemiol.* 2003, 158(6), 503-8.
[17]   Schimmel, MS; Eidelman, AI; Zadka, P; Kornbluth, E; Hammerman,
        C. Increased parity and risk of trisomy 21: review of 37,110 live births.
        BMJ. 1997, 314, 720–1.
[18]   Dolan, SM; Callaghan, WM; Rasmussen, SA. Birth defects and
        preterm birth: overlapping outcomes with a shared strategy for research
        and prevention. *Birth Defects Res. A Clin. Mol. Teratol.* 2009
        Nov;85(11):874-8
[19]   Honein, MA; Kirby, RS; Meyer, RE; Xing, J; Skerrette, NI; Yuskiv, N;
        Marengo, L; Petrini, JR; Davidoff, MJ; Mai, CT; Druschel, CM; Viner-
        Brown, S; Sever, LE; National Birth Defects Prevention Network. The
        association between major birth defects and preterm birth. *Matern.
        Child Health J.* 2009 Mar;13(2):164-75. Epub 2008 May 17.
[20]   American College of Obstetricians and Gynecologists (ACOG). 2000.
        Planning your pregnancy. American College of Obstetricians and
        Gynecologists, Washington, DC.

[21]   March of Dimes (MOD). 2009. March of Dimes. Available at: www. marchofdimes.com. Accessed 27 September 2009.

[22]   Glinianaia, SV; Rankin, J; Wright, C. Congenital anomalies in twins: a register-based study. *Hum. Reprod.* 2008, 23(6), 1306-11.

[23]   Pharoah, PO; Glinianaia, SV; Rankin, J. Congenital anomalies in multiple births after early loss of a conceptus. *Hum. Reprod.* 2009, 24(3), 726-31.

[24]   Harman, CR. Amniotic fluid abnormalities. *Semin. Perinatol.* 2008 Aug;32(4):288-94.

[25]   Noronha Neto, C; Souza, AS; Moraes Filho, OB; Noronha, AM. Amniotic fluid volume associated with fetal anomalies diagnosed in a reference center in the Brazilian Northeast. *Rev. Bras. Ginecol. Obstet.* 2009 Apr;31(4):164-70.

[26]   Monk, D; Moore GE. Intrauterine growth restriction--genetic causes and consequences. *Semin. Fetal Neonatal. Med.* 2004 Oct;9(5):371-8.

[27]   Hendrix, N; Berghella V. Non-placental causes of intrauterine growth restriction. *Semin. Perinatol.* 2008 Jun;32(3):161-5.

[28]   Vora, N; Bianchi DW. Genetic considerations in the prenatal diagnosis of overgrowth syndromes. *Prenat. Diagn.* 2009 Oct;29(10):923-9.

[29]   Waller, DK; Keddie, AM; Canfield, MA; Scheuerle, AE. Do infants with major congenital anomalies have an excess of macrosomia? *Teratology.* 2001 Dec;64(6):311-7.

[30]   Kaplan, M; Hammerman, C. Understanding severe hyperbilirubinemia and preventing kernicterus: adjuncts in the interpretation of neonatal serum bilirubin. *Clin. Chim. Acta.* 2005 Jun;356(1-2):9-21.

[31]   Bertini, G; Dani, C; Pezzati, M; Rubaltelli, FF. Prevention of bilirubin encephalopathy. *Biol. Neonate.* 2001;79(3-4):219-23.

[32]   Subcommittee on Hyperbilirubinemia, American Academy of Pediatrics. Clinical Practice Guideline: management of hyperbilirubinemia in the newborn infant 35 or more weeks of gestation. *Pediatrics.* 2004;114:297–316.

[33]   Crane, JM; van den Hof, MC; Dodds, L; Armson, BA; Liston, R. Neonatal outcomes with placenta previa. *Obstet. Gynecol.* 1999 Apr;93(4):541-4.

[34]   Sheiner, E; Shoham-Vardi, I; Hallak, M; Hershkowitz, R; Katz, M; Mazor, M. Placenta previa: obstetric risk factors and pregnancy outcome. *J. Matern. Fetal. Med.* 2001 Dec;10(6):414-9.

[35]   Vesce, F; Farina, A; Giorgetti, M; Jorizzo, G; Bianciotto, A; Calabrese, O; Mollica, G. Increased incidence of preeclampsia in pregnancies

complicated by fetal malformation. *Gynecol. Obstet. Invest.* 1997;44(2):107-11.

[36]   Presler, JL. Classification of major newborn birth injuries. *J. Perinat. Neonatal Nurs.* 2008 Jan-Mar;22(1):60-7.

[37]   Levine, MG; Holroyde, J; Woods, JR ; Siddiqi, TA; Scott, M; Miodovnik, M. Birth trauma: incidence and predisposing factors. *Obstet. Gynecol.* 1984 Jun;63(6):792-5.

[38]   Ortibus, E. Early and long-term consequences of intrapartum asphyxia. International Congress Series Volume 1279, April 2005, Pages 353-357

[39]   Zupan Simunek, V. Definition of intrapartum asphyxia and effects on outcome. *J. Gynecol. Obstet. Biol. Reprod.* (Paris). 2008 Feb;37 Suppl 1:S7-15.

[40]   Wu, YW; Colford JM Jr. Chorioamnionitis as a risk factor for cerebral palsy: A meta-analysis. *JAMA.* 2000 Sep 20;284(11):1417-

Chapter III

Maternal Health Conditions

More subtle genetic effects that more obviously involve the environment as well occur through some maternal illnesses. Maternal health conditions that contribute to increased risks for congenital anomalies include many diseases such as diabetes mellitus, epilepsy controlled with anticonvulsant medications, phenylketonuria, thyroid diseases, deep vein thrombosis, depression and other mental disorders [1,2].

Diagnosis and treatment of any chronic diseases in women such as anemia and urinary tract infection before pregnancy is also very important for the pregnancy outcomes.

Diabetes Mellitus (DM)

Insulin-dependent diabetes mellitus (DM) is a multifactorial disease. If a pregnant mother has this disease and it is not well controlled, an unfavourable environment for the developing embryo arises, and malformations may occur. The severity of the defects is related to the level of diabetic control [2]. Nongenetic structural anomalies in the offspring of women with prepregnancy DM are likely attributable to an embryonic insult before seven weeks after gestation [3].

Major and minor congenital anomalies affect together between 5-10% of fetuses born to women with type 1 DM, a rate approximately 5-10 times higher than that in the non diabetic population. Major anomalies, causing death or serious handicap necessitating surgical correction or medical therapy, include those of the central nervous (e.g anencephaly and spina bifida), cardiac (e.g transposition of the great vessels, atrial and ventrikular septal defects), and genitourinary (e.g. renal dysgenesis, duplex ureters). Diabetes mellitus in pregnant mothers is a risk factor for neural tube defects (NTDs). The risk for NTDs in diabetic pregnancy is two to fivefold higher than in normal, non-diabetic pregnancy [3,4,5,6].

Such malformations are associated with poor blood glucose control before and during pregnancy. Preconception care in women with diabetes is essential to reduce these and improve the outcome of subsequent pregnancies. Pregnancy-related advice should be offered to all girls with diabetes starting during puberty. Screening for high-risk delivery, health promotion and effective interventions should be carried out by a multidisciplinary team that includes a diabetologist or endocrinologist, nurse as diabetes educators, an obstetrician and a dietitian. For women with diabetes, preconception care ideally begins between 3 and 6 months before conception. Optimized pre-conception care is based on a comprehensive assessment of a woman's entire medical history together with a physical examination, and an evaluation of risk factors, family history, medications, and dietary and exercise habits. An assessment of diabetes in preconception care should also focus on metabolic control and HbA_{1c}, vascular and lipid status, renal function, and should include an electrocardiogram, a fundoscopic examination and tests of thyroid function [5,6,7,8].

A complete physical assessment should include blood pressure measurements, a retinal examination and, if needed, a follow-up examination at the end of the first trimester of pregnancy, neurological assessments, a lower-extremity examination, and a pelvic examination, including pap smear. Achieving good blood glucose control is important in the first trimester in order to avoid fetal malformation and hyperglycemic complications. The International Diabetes Federation (IDF) [9] global guideline for type 2 diabetes recommends the preconception target of HbA_{1c} lower than 6.1%; the American Diabetes Association (ADA) [10] guideline recommends HbA_{1c} below 7% before conception is attempted. For women who have not met treatment goals, education and the initiation of blood glucose self-monitoring are also necessary. Women with type 2 diabetes using oral blood glucose-lowering medications should begin insulin therapy.

Good blood glucose control before conception and throughout pregnancy will reduce the risk of malformation, stillbirth and neonatal death. Strict metabolic control well before conception and educating the women about the risk of diabetes mellitus can significantly reduce the incidence of birth defects among infants of diabetic mothers. Optimization of glycemic control before pregnancy, in conjunction with other PCC interventions, may lead to a 65% average relative risk reduction in major congenital anomalies [3]. Clinical trials have demonstrated that preconception care and glycemic control can lower considerably the rate of congenital malformations in the offspring of diabetic mothers. These studies, which explored the influence of pre-conception normoglycemia and post-conception strict metabolic control on prevalence of major congenital anomalies, revealed positive results (reduction in the incidence of major congenital anomalies). The combination of the results of the prospective studies reveals a malformation rate of ~2% among the offspring of preconception registered and treated mothers, and 10% for the postconception group [4].

Counseling should include about the risk and prevention of congenital anomalies; fetal and neonatal complications of maternal diabetes; effects of pregnancy on maternal diabetic complications; risks of obstetrical complications that occur with increased frequency in diabetic pregnancies (especially hypertensive disorders); the need for effective contraception until glycemia is wellcontrolled; and the cost-benefit relationship between preconception care and prevention of malformations [11].

Recommended steps as part of prepregnancy counseling in women with type 1 or type 2 DM; [3]

1. Explain risks of congenital anomalies and probable risk reduction with optimal glycemic control
2. Assess current medications and need to stop
3. Encourage self-measurement and written recording of capillary blood glucose concentrations 2–4 times/day
4. Encourage use of insulin injections twice daily (for type 2 DM) or four times daily (for type 1 DM) to achieve premeal (fasting) glucose concentrations of 4–7 mmol/l
5. Suggest having a nonperishable glucose source on self, as well as in automobile and at bedside to deal with early hypoglycemia
6. Encourage use of effective contraception (i.e., oral contraceptive pill or condom with spermicide) until glycemic control optimized
7. Encourage use of oral folic acid, 1 mg daily
8. Encourage smoking cessation
9. Obtain baseline glycosylated hemoglobin concentration

10. Refer to a diabetes education center and/or specialist (e.g. endocrinologist)

Epilepsy

The prevalence of epilepsy is 0.4-1.0 % in the general population; about 25% of these patients are women of childbearing years. Every year, about 0.3–0.4 % of all children is born to mothers with epilepsy. It is commonly known that there is a 2- to 3-fold increased prevalence of major and minor malformations in the offspring of epileptic women compared to the general population. These abnormalities can largely be attributed to the teratogenic effects of antiepileptic drugs (AEDs). However, the maternal epilepsy itself could also play a role because of the genetic risks that may go together with the maternal disease. The transplacental metabolic effects of the maternal disease and the impairment of fetoplacental circulation due to maternal seizures also have to be taken into account. Epileptic women face the problem of balancing the teratogenic risks resulting from seizures during pregnancy against the risks of taking AEDs to prevent these seizures. Therefore knowledge and prevention of AED-related abnormalities are important factors in the care of epileptic women and their offspring [12,13].

Antiepileptic drugs, as a class, are widely known to be associated with congenital anomalies and, unlike other medications, in patients with active epilepsy they generally cannot be discontinued, even when pregnancy is planned. As a result, adverse effects on fetuses are a major concern for millions of women with epilepsy, and the physicians responsible for their care [14]. Overall, AEDs have been associated with an increased risk of major congenital malformations, minor anomalies, specific congenital syndromes, and developmental disorders seen in childhood. However, the differential effects of individual AEDs remain uncertain. Data are accumulating which strongly suggest that these risks are highest in patients receiving polypharmacy and valproate. There is also modest evidence to suggest an increased risk for phenobarbital. While other older AEDs appear to carry some teratogenic risk, there is not adequate evidence to further stratify their risk [15]. Maternal teratogenic effects cannot be separated from the teratogenic effect of medication. Anti-epileptic drugs (AED) cross the placenta, raise the pharmacologically active concentration of the drug in the embryo or fetus, alter folate metabolism, and decrease the plasma folate or red-cell folate concentration. Although the mechanisms underlying the effects of AED have yet to be elucidated in detail, several theories have been suggested for their adverse effects, such as liver enzyme induction by AED, the impairment of folate absorption, competitive interaction between folate co-enzymes and drugs, and an increased demand for folate as a co-enzyme for antiepileptic hydroxylation. The drugs were associated with heart defects, clept lip and clept palate, and, to a lesser extent, with major malformations like skeletal abnormalities, whereas closure defects of the neural tube were relatively rare. Growth and psychomotor development are additional important end points of teratogenesis. Women with epilepsy who could become pregnant should be given supplementation with 0·4–5·0 mg/day folic acid, with some authors recommending doses of 4 mg/day or 5 mg/day only for women taking valproic acid and carbamazepine or otherwise at high risk for neural tube defects [14,16].

Prevention of abnormalities pregnancy outcome is an important aspect of the care of women with epilepsy, before and during pregnancy, and after delivery. Primary prevention aims at reducing the teratogenic risks by obtaining complete seizure control with the least amount of teratogenic medication. Management of women with epilepsy should involve avoidance of valproic acid (particularly high-dose valproic acid) when suitable alternatives are available, avoidance of unnecessary polytherapy, prophylactic treatment with folic acid, and counseling about contraception and discussion of the risks in pregnancy [12,14,15].

If the maternal epilepsy necessitates medication that is associated with an increased risk of specific malformations, prenatal diagnosis may be offered including appropriate ultrasound investigations. Etiology of the epilepsy, type, severity and frequency of seizures and EEG abnormalities all play a role in treatment decision [12]. The benefits of AEDs in suppressing seizures should not be underestimated, and the dangers of abrupt discontinuation of treatment, including status epilepticus and seizure-associated maternal mortality, should be highlighted. Because seizures may harm both the mother and the fetus, and because most major congenital anomalies are likely to have already occurred when pregnancy is diagnosed, treatment changes during pregnancy should only be made if required for seizure control [14].

Phenylketonuria

Phenylketonuria (PKU) is a purely genetic condition, being inherited in an autosomal recessive manner. The enzyme phenylalanine hydroxylase is absent, and unless controlled by a special diet, excess phenylalanine accumulates in the blood. This is toxic, especially to the brain, and irreversible mental retardation results. If an affected woman is untreated in pregnancy, the excess phenylalanine reaches the embryonic environment. As a result, and even if, as is usual, the baby is genotypically normal, the phenylalanine-rich environment will produce embryopathy. Maternal phenylketonuria embryopathy includes microcephaly, mental retardation, congenital heart disease, facial dysmorphism and intrauterine growth retardation [2,17,18].

Diet has long been recognized as the primary treatment modality for individuals with PKU during infancy and childhood. Well-established dietary protocols have prevented mental retardation for infants born with PKU. Dietary protocols for managing females with PKU in their reproductive years exist but are not followed by most of them [17]. Recent findings from the Maternal PKU Collaborative Study clearly indicate that dietary restriction of phenylalanine is also necessary to prevent the adverse effects of an elevated plasma phenylalanine concentration during pregnancy. A women with PKU should closely adhere to a low- phenylalanine diet before conception to avoid build up of toxic metabolic products in her body that may damage the fetus [16,19].

The aims of management are to maintain blood phenylalanine concentration in the target range (100–250 μmol/L) before and throughout the pregnancy, and to ensure adequate maternal nutrition and appropriate weight gain. Blood phenylalanine is monitored twice, three times a week, before and after conception respectively. Weight is monitored on a weekly basis and key micronutrients are monitored every 6–8 weeks in clinic. From the second trimester onwards, dietary phenylalanine intake has to be promptly increased, as phenylalanine tolerance increases rapidly. Postnatal management includes a neurological assessment of the infant at 4–8 weeks and an echocardiogram for infants conceived off diet. Subsequently, offspring are seen at 1 year, 4 years, 8 years and 14 years for neuropsychometric evaluations. Regular follow-up of the mother remains important whether on or off a phenylalanine-restricted diet [20].

In a study investigated the role of nutrition in pregnancy with phenylketonuria and birth defects, the data indicated that blood Phe control and how soon it is attained during pregnancy with PKU is important. Normal pregnancy weight gain should be encouraged to reduce microcephaly. Adequate protein and vitamin intakes early in pregnancy may have a protective effect for the prevention of congenital heart disease, even if blood Phe is elevated. The rate of microcephaly and congenital heart disease may be reduced if nutrient intake is optimal while attempting to control blood Phe levels [21].

Physicians, advanced practice nurses (APNs), and metabolic dietitians taking care of females with PKU should routinely discuss PKU pregnancy and the potential for severe birth defects during clinic visits [17]. Healthcare providers managing pregnant women (obstetricians, family practitioners, midwives) must be made aware of the risk indicators and potential severe fetal morbidity (and medico-legal implications) of a missed cases including undiagnosed or lost to follow-up maternal PKU patients. In addition practitioners caring for infants with any of the stigmata of Maternal PKU embryopathy must remember to test the mothers for PKU to prevent damage to future fetuses [18].

Biochemical newborn screening to detect phenylketonuria is an established method of secondary prevention of birth defects in the developed world [22]. The system was introduced in the 1960's for phenylketonuria, because a low phenylalanine diet prevents severe mental retardation if started in the first weeks of life [23].

Women with PKU and their families require much psychosocial support to meet the strict requirements of a maternal PKU pregnancy, including compliance with a difficult diet. With such compliance, however, it seems that bearing normal or near normal offspring is possible [24].

Thyroid Diseases

Thyroid diseases in pregnancy must be recognized as a specific challenge. Any pregnancy is causing alterations in thyroid hormone metabolism which have to be differentiated from pathologic states of thyroid function. Any thyroid disease of the mother with disturbances in the functional state of the gland could induce an adverse influence on the course of pregnancy. Furthermore, it can be associated with adverse consequences on fetal development [25]. Abnormalities of maternal thyroid function can affect the fetus directly or indirectly. The fetal thyroid begins to produce thyroid hormones after the first trimester, so the critical thyroid hormones for fetal brain development must be supplied by the mother [26]. Especially hypothyroidism has to be avoided during pregnancy due to a danger of affected neurocognitive development of the offspring. Yet also maternal hyperthyroidism can lead to impairments in the course of pregnancy and to fetal thyroid dysfunction [25].

Hypothyroidism

The prevalence of hypothyroidism during pregnancy is estimated to be 0.3 − 0.5% for overt hypothyroidism and 2 − 3% for subclinical hypothyroidism. Overall, the most common cause of hypothyroidism is the autoimmune disorder known as Hashimoto's thyroiditis. Hypothyroidism can occur during pregnancy due to the initial presentation of Hashimoto's thyroiditis, inadequate treatment of a woman already known to have hypothyroidism from a variety of causes, or over-treatment of a hyperthyroid woman with anti-thyroid medications. Other causes of hypothyroidism include radioiodine ablation of the thyroid, thyroidectomy, and noncompliance with existing levothyroxine (LT4) therapy [26,27,28].

Maternal hypothyroidism is correlated with neurodevelopmental deficits in children, with the severity of the deficit directly related to the severity of the thyroid deficiency [29]. Effects of hypothyroidism on the fetus include fetal abnormalities, low birth weight, perinatal mortality, neonatal morbidity, and impaired neurocognitive development. During the first-half of gestation when fetal brain development occurs, fetal T4 is derived primarily from the mother. Therefore, maternal hypothyroidism has the greatest impact on fetal neurodevelopment during the first and second trimesters [28].

It is reported that, maternal thyroid hormone levels in pregnancy have been linked to childhood neurodevelopmental level, including motor findings. Maternal FT4 concentration below the 10th percentile at 12 weeks of gestation significantly increased the risk for impaired motor development by 5.8-fold [30]. A significant delay was found in mental and motor development for 1-years-olds and 2-years-olds born to the women with hypothyroxinaemia before 12 weeks (FT4 < 10th and TSH within reference range: 0.15 − 2 mU/l), but if hypothyroxinaemia was established after the 12th week of gestation no impaired development was found [26].

Thyroid hormone is critical for brain development in the baby. Children born with congenital hypothyroidism (no thyroid function at birth) can have severe cognitive, neurological and developmental abnormalities if the condition is not recognized and treated promptly. These developmental abnormalities can largely be prevented if the disease is recognized and treated immediately after birth [27].

The diagnosis of hypothyroidism during pregnancy is crucial because of its potential adverse effects on the mother and child that can be prevented with adequate therapy. There are indications that the children of women with hypothyroidism untreated until after the first trimester may suffer from impairment in final intellectual and cognitive abilities. Thereafter, despite thyroxin therapy, nobody can reassure parents about potential brain damage of the children if longstanding intrauterine hypothyroidism has been present [26].

Endocrine Society clinical practice guideline [31] have recommended following interventions for the management of hypothyroidism during pregnancy and postpartum:

- If hypothyroidism has been diagnosed before pregnancy, the guideline panel recommends adjustment of the preconception thyroxine dose to reach before pregnancy a thyroid-stimulating hormone (TSH) level not higher than 2.5 mIU/liter.
- The thyroxine dose often needs to be incremented by 4 to 6 weeks gestation and may require a 30 to 50% increment in dosage.
- If diagnosed during pregnancy, thyroid function tests should be normalized as rapidly as possible. Thyroxine dosage should be titrated to rapidly reach and thereafter maintain serum TSH concentrations of less than 2.5 mI/liter in the first trimester (or 3 mIU/liter in second and third trimesters) or to trimester-specific normal TSH ranges. Thyroid function tests should be premeasured within 30 to 40 days.
- Women with thyroid autoimmunity who are euthyroid in the early stages of pregnancy are at risk of developing hypothyroidism and should be monitored for elevation of TSH above the normal range.
- Subclinical hypothyroidism (serum TSH concentration above the upper limit of the reference range with a normal free T4) has been shown to be associated with an adverse outcome for both the mother and offspring. Thyroxine treatment has been shown to improve obstetrical outcome, but has not been proved to modify long-term neurological development in the offspring. However, given that the potential benefits outweigh the potential risks, the panel recommends thyroxine replacement in women with subclinical hypothyroidism.
- After delivery, most hypothyroid women need to decrease the thyroxine dosage they received during pregnancy

Hyperthyroidism

The prevalence of hyperthyroidism during pregnancy is approximately 0.2%, with most cases being due to Graves' disease. Overall, the most common cause (80-85%) of maternal hyperthyroidism during pregnancy is

Graves' disease and occurs in 1 in 1500 pregnant patients. In addition to other usual causes of hyperthyroidism, very high levels of hCG, seen in severe forms of morning sickness (*hyperemesis gravidarum*), may cause transient hyperthyroidism [27,28].

Uncontrolled maternal hyperthyroidism has been associated with fetal tachycardia, low birth weight, prematurity, intrauterine growth retardation, stillbirths and possibly congenital malformations. Although uncommon (2-5% of cases of Graves' disease in pregnancy), high levels of maternal thyroid stimulating immunoglobulins (TSI's), have been known to cause fetal or neonatal hyperthyroidism. Treatment of the hyperthyroid state decreases these complications [27,28].

When comparing children born to mothers with and without elevated serum TSH in mid-gestation, effects on cognition were seen. Infants born to mothers with TSH levels in the upper 2% of the population had 4.7 the odds of having an IQ one SD below the population mean. Such IQ levels were found in 5% of controls, but in 19% of exposed children. Also it was found that the mothers of children with cerebral palsy were more likely to have been diagnosed with hyperthyroidism before pregnancy and to have received thyroid hormone treatment during pregnancy [30].

The diagnosis of hyperthyroidism can be somewhat difficult during pregnancy, as ^{123}I thyroid scanning is contraindicated during pregnancy due to the small amount of radioactivity, which can be concentrated by the baby's thyroid. Consequently, diagnosis is based on a careful history, physical exam and laboratory testing [27].

Radioactive iodine is a highly efficacious therapy for hyperthyroidism. However, use of radioactive iodine is contraindicated in pregnancy because iodine crosses the placenta and exposes the fetal thyroid. When a pregnant woman inadvertently receives a therapeutic dose of radioiodine as iodine-131 (I131) the risk to the fetus is significant and can include ablation of the fetal thyroid, mental retardation, malformations, growth changes, induction of malignancies, and fetal loss. The outcome depends on the gestational age at which exposure occurs. If radioiodine exposure occurs when the fetal thyroid is capable of trapping iodine, there is a definite risk of subsequent fetal hypothyroidism. Congenital hypothyroidism has been reported in offspring of mothers who received therapeutic doses of radioiodine. Other outcomes such as spontaneous abortions, stillbirth, biliary atresia, respiratory distress, and mental deficiency have been described [28].

Endocrine Society clinical practice guideline [31] have recommended following interventions for the management of hyperthyroidism during pregnancy and postpartum:

- Because available evidence suggests that methimazole (MMI) may be associated with congenital anomalies, propylthiouracil (PTU) should be used as a first-line drug, if available, especially during first-trimester organogenesis. MMI may be prescribed if propylthiouracil is not available, or if a patient cannot tolerate or has an adverse response to propylthiouracil.
- Subtotal thyroidectomy may be indicated during pregnancy as therapy for maternal Graves' disease if 1) a patient has a severe adverse reaction to antithyroid drug- ATD therapy, 2) persistently high doses of ATD are required, or 3) a patient is nonadherent to ATD therapy and has uncontrolled hyperthyroidism. The optimal timing of surgery is in the second trimester.
- There is no evidence that treatment of subclinical hyperthyroidism improves pregnancy outcome, and treatment could potentially adversely affect fetal outcome.
- Because thyroid receptor antibodies (thyroid receptor stimulating, binding, or inhibiting antibodies) freely cross the placenta and can stimulate the fetal thyroid, these antibodies should be measured by the end of the second trimester in mothers with current Graves' disease or with a history of Graves' disease and treatment with 131-I or thyroidectomy before pregnancy, or with a previous neonate with Graves' disease. Women who have a negative TSH-receptor antibody (TRAb) and do not require antithyroid drug ATD have a very low risk of fetal or neonatal thyroid dysfunction.
- 131-I should not be given to a woman who is or may be pregnant. If inadvertently treated, the patient should be promptly informed of the radiation danger to the fetus, including thyroid destruction if treated after the 12th week of gestation.
- In women with elevated TRAb or in women treated with ATD, fetal ultrasound should be performed to look for evidence of fetal thyroid dysfunction, which could include growth restriction, hydrops, presence of goiter, advanced bone age, or cardiac failure.
- Umbilical blood sampling should be considered only if the diagnosis of fetal thyroid disease is not reasonably certain from the clinical data and the information gained would change the treatment.

- All newborns of mothers with Graves' disease should be evaluated by a medical care provider for thyroid dysfunction and treated if necessary.

Mental Illness

Depression and other mood disorders are common during pregnancy, with an estimated prevalence ranging from 9% to 16% [32]. While the prevalence of serious mental illness such as schizophrenia remains low, it is estimated that up to one in 5 women will experience clinically diagnosable depression or anxiety during pregnancy and the postpartum period [33,34].

Choosing the right treatment for a pregnant or breastfeeding woman with a mood or anxiety disorder is a difficult task given the uncertainty surrounding the potential risks of medication. The common concern for many pregnant women is whether a medication will affect the development of their child, and in the absence of reassuring information, many will either forgo necessary pharmacotherapy or cease existing treatment, much to their own and that of their child's detriment [35]. Untreated psychiatric illness poses dangers to both mother and child, while discontinuation of psychotropic medication poses its own hazards. Management therefore calls for a balanced risk-benefit analysis of the mother and fetus/neonate along with careful review of the most recent research evidence. Several factors must be considered, including possible teratogenic effects of medication, the safety of medication during labor and delivery, possible long-term neurobehavioral effects and the effects of ongoing exposure during breastfeeding [36]. Consequently, treating a psychiatric disorder during pregnancy with pharmacotherapy, is a complex decision making process, which has to be made between the pregnant woman and her health care provider [37].

A discussion about teratogenicity from the medication, even if the risk is viewed as small in comparison to the risks of the untreated mental illness, may provoke concern in most expectant mothers. Treatment selection is influenced by:

- illness factors such as severity of symptoms
- relevant past history and effective treatments
- time interval between previous cessation of medication and relapse of the disorder and level of functioning in this interval
- the likelihood of compliance

- suicide risk
- the risks to the infant, including potential for neglect, and parental concerns around the medication, and financial and time constraints.

It is important to consider both pharmacological and nonpharmacological approaches to the management of a woman with mental illness during the pregnancy and postpartum period treatment, much to their own and that of their child's detriment [35].

Preconception planning is perhaps the ideal scenario, and achievable theoretically by offering prophylactic advice to all female psychiatric patients of childbearing age. In addition to providing the patient valuable information relevant to the implications of their pathology (and its treatment) on the unborn child, this approach allows the exploration of non-pharmacological control of the mental state prior to conception and during pregnancy, thus minimizing exposure of the unborn child to potentially teratogenic medication [36]. The importance of preconception counseling is crucial but often opportunistic. The window of opportunity may be missed by an unplanned pregnancy or late presentation. Even if the 'horse has bolted', postconception counseling can be beneficial [33].

Drug treatment is indicated if psychotherapy is inadequate or inappropriate for the patient's severity of illness. Once a decision to offer pharmacotherapy is made, important factors in drug selection for the mother include efficacy of the drugs available, the anticipated response of the individual patient, and the overall toxicity profile of the drug for the mother and fetus. Potential adverse effects for the fetus and the neonate include:

1) structural malformations,
2) acute neonatal effects including intoxication and neonatal abstinence syndromes,
3) intrauterine fetal death,
4) altered fetal growth, and
5) neurobehavioral teratogenicity [38].

Antenatal exposure to psychotropic agents carries the risks of teratogenicity, toxicity and possible long-term neurobehavioural problems. Maternal medication during the first trimester of pregnancy, particularly between the third and eighth weeks of gestation, is most relevant with regard to morphological teratogenesis, whilst that during the second and third trimesters may have deleterious effects on growth and/or functional development and toxic effects. Despite the risks to the fetus associated with medication during pregnancy, an unacceptably high risk of deterioration of the mental state often mandates continued psychotropic medication. When such risk outweighs the risks of medication to the fetus, the minimum therapy consistent with control of psychiatric disease should be prescribed. It may also be worth exploring the option of withholding medication (or reducing the dose thereof) until after the first trimester with a view to protecting the fetus from potentially teratogenic stimuli during this essential phase of organogenesis, although this carries the risk of recurrence of psychiatric disease [36].

Data published mainly before 2000 and obtained from small teratology information service databases supported the lack of an association between use of SSRIs (selective serotonin reuptake inhibitors) during pregnancy and an increased risk for development of major malformations. However, more recent data from large population-based studies using more appropriate pharmacoepidemiologic approaches have challenged this assumption. Recent guidelines and updated teratogenic classifications recommend cautious use of SSRIs during pregnancy and avoidance of paroxetine. Paroxetine was the first SSRI to be associated with an enhanced risk of birth defects, particularly cardiac defects. Similar concerns do not appear to apply to other SSRIs, despite recent findings suggesting a certain degree of risk with other SSRIs, particularly fluoxetine [32,39]. Infants exposed in utero to an SSRI in combination with a benzodiazepine may have a higher a incidence of congenital heart defects compared to no exposure, even after controlling for maternal illness characteristics [34].

Mood stabilizers such as lithium and sodium valproate are highly problematic if used during pregnancy and present major challenges in managing the pregnant woman with bipolar affective disorder. Lithium is reported to produce congenital cardiovascular malformations (especially Ebstein's anomaly) in the fetus when used in the first trimester. However recent reevaluation of this risk concludes that Ebstein's anomaly is rare and the risk is much lower than originally reported [33,36,38].

The fetal hydantoin syndrome consisting of facial dysmorphism, cleft lip and palate, cardiac defects, digital hypoplasia, and nail dysplasia was initially ascribed to the use of phenytoin during pregnancy. It is now recognized to occur with carbamazepine and valproic acid as well. NTDs also are associated with carbamazepine and valproic acid [38].

Sodium valproate usage in the first trimester is associated with a rate of up to 20% for serious adverse outcomes, including malformation. Sodium valproate exposure has also been associated with neurodevelopmental abnormalities in the unborn child with continued use throughout the pregnancy. Valproic acid is associated with a variety of congenital malformations. The prevalence of neural tube defects/spina bifida is reportedly 1–2%, a tenfold increase. Other abnormalities include malformations of the limbs and digits, the urogenital tract, the heart and cerebral dysfunction evidenced by psychomotor tardiness, neurological dysfunction and hyperexcitability. Craniofacial anomalies and low birth weight have also been reported. Doses in excess of 1,000 mg per day and the use of multiple anticonvulsants appear to increase the risk of congenital malformations [33,36].

Carbamazepine is also problematic and lamotrigine has been associated with an increased risk of oral clefts. Carbamazepine is recognized as teratogenic, though perhaps less so than valproic acid. A 0.5–1.0% risk of spina bifida, microcephaly, craniofacial anomalies, cardiovascular anomalies, urogenital malformations and growth retardation has been reported. [33,36].

Tricyclic antidepressants are relatively safe. The majority of published data suggest that tricyclic antidepressants (TCAs) appear to be free of teratogenic risk. Insufficient human data exist to ascertain the teratogenicity of monamine oxidase inhibitors. Commencement of these drugs during pregnancy is therefore not advisable; indeed it is recommended that women already on Monoamine oxidase inhibitors MAOIs should ideally be switched to alternative agents preferably prior to conception, or immediately upon diagnosis of pregnancy [36,38,39]

The belief that diazepan causes congenital malformations, especially cleft lip/palate, is controversial. Caution is advised with the use of benzodiazepines in pregnancy [33,36,39].

Table 1. Maternal Diseases, Congenital Anomalies and Prevention

Maternal Disease	Congenital Anomaly	Prevention
Diabetes mellitus (DM) – associated with poor blood glucose control before and during pregnancy	– central nervous system (anencephaly and spina bifida, neural tube defects (NTDs). – cardiac (e.g transposition of the great vessels, atrial and ventrikular septal defects), – genitourinary (renal dysgenesis, duplex ureters).	– Pre-conception care – glycemic control HbA$_{1c}$ below 7% before conception – prophylactic treatment with folic acid
Epilepsy – teratogenic effects of antiepileptic drugs – metabolic effects of the maternal disease – impaired fetoplacental circulation due to maternal seizures	– heart defects, – clept lip and clept palate, – skeletal abnormalities, – neural tube closure defects o – growth and psychomotor development	– the least amount of teratogenic medication – avoidance of valproic acid – prophylactic treatment with folic acid
Phenylketonuria (PKU) – toxic effects of excess phenylalanine	– microcephaly, – mental retardation, – congenital heart disease, – facial dysmorphism – IUGR	– low- phenylalanine diet before conception – Normal pregnancy weight gain – Biochemical newborn screening

Maternal Disease	Congenital Anomaly	Prevention
Hypothyroidism – Low maternal thyroid hormone levels in pregnancy	– neurodevelopmental deficits – cognitive, neurological and developmental problems	– thyroxin therapy before and during
Hyperthyroidism – High maternal thyroid hormone levels in pregnancy	– fetal or neonatal hyperthyroidism – cognitive abnormalities	– radioactive iodine is contraindicated in pregnancy – antithyroid drug therapy
Mental Illness – teratogenic effects of psychotherapy	– structural malformations – neurodevelopmental abnormalities – cardiac defects – Ebstein's anomaly	– avoidance of medication where possible, especially during the first trimester – the minimum therapy for the control of psychiatric disease – avoidance of valproic acid, carbamazepine, hydantoin, MAOIs – caution with benzodiazepines, SSRI's, lithium – folic acid supplementation

General principles for use of medication; [33]

- Medication should be avoided where possible, especially during the first trimester; however untreated mental illness also poses risks during this time
- Following consultation, an agreed plan, with appropriate input from the woman, her partner, the general practitioner, the obstetrician and the psychiatrist, is followed
- If conception occurs unexpectedly, medication should not be withdrawn abruptly; medical guidance is necessary
- If medication is used an effective dose should be prescribed. Generally, the principle of 'start slow, go slow' applies
- Monotherapy up to therapeutic or higher doses is preferred over combination therapy
- If a medication has been effective in the past this should be the first choice
- Careful monitoring, especially during periods of change, is essential
- Adequate folic acid supplementation (5 mg) needs to be considered, especially with certain medication (e.g. anticonvulsants)
- In patients with a history of severe mental illness, prophylaxis can be considered in late pregnancy
- Medication used in pregnancy should be continued postpartum
- Neonatal discontinuation symptoms are not uncommon, although rarely severe. The infant may need to be monitored closely for the first 5 days
- Information changes rapidly and it is important to keep up-to-date

When there is a history of severe mental illness such as a past history of psychosis or psychiatric hospitalization, or multiple medications and complex health care needs, early specialist involvement is indicated. In these vulnerable women, it is important to maintain consistency and continuity of care with close liaison between obstetric, mental health services and the general practitioner [33]. Optimal control of the psychiatric disorder should be maintained during pregnancy, the post partum period and thereafter. All pregnancies where a mother has a serious psychiatric disorder should be considered high risk and the mother and fetus must be carefully monitored [37]

References

[1]   Health Canada. Congenital Anomalies in Canada — A Perinatal Health Report, 2002. Ottawa: Minister of Public Works and Government Services Canada, 2002.

[2]   Seller, M. Genetic Causes of Congenital Anomalies and Their Interaction with Environmental Factors. In: EUROCAT Special Report. The environmental causes of congenital anomalies: a review of the literature. www.eurocat.ulster.ac.uk/pubdata

[3]   McLeod, L; Ray, JG. Prevention and detection of diabetic embryopathy. *Community Genet.* 2002;5(1), 33-9.

[4]   Eriksson, UJ. Congenital anomalies in diabetic pregnancy. *Semin. Fetal Neonatal. Med.* 2009, 14(2), 85-93.

[5]   Garne, E. Maternal Diabetes. In: EUROCAT Special Report. The environmental causes of congenital anomalies: a review of the literature.

[6]   Ozcan, S; Sahin, N. Reproductive health in women with diabetes: The need for pre-conception care and education, *Diabetes Voices,* 2009, 54, special issue: 21-24.

[7]   Canadian Diabetes Association. 2008 Clinical Practice Guidelines. Canadian Journal of Diabetes, 2008, 32 (Suppl 1).

[8]   National Collaborating Centre for Women's and Children's Health. Diabetes in pregnancy: management of diabetes and its complications from pre-conception to the postnatal period. RCOG Press at the Royal College of Obstetricians and Gynaecologists. London, 2008. (www.nice.org.uk/CG063fullguideline)

[9]   International Diabetes Federation. Global Guideline for Type 2 Diabetes. IDF. Brussels, 2005.

[10]   American Diabetes Association. Standards of Medical Care in Diabetes. *Diabetes Care.* 2009, 32(Suppl 1).

[11]   American Diabetes Association. Preconception Care Of Women With Diabetes. Position Statement. *Diabetes Care.* Volume 26, Supplement 1, January 2003

[12]   Berg, KT; Lindhout, D. Antiepileptic Drugs in pregnancy, Community Genet, 2002, 5, 40-49.

[13]   Robert, E. Maternal Epilepsy. In: EUROCAT Special Report. The environmental causes of congenital anomalies: a review of the literature. www.eurocat.ulster.ac.uk/pubdata

[14]   Perucca, E. Birth defects after prenatal exposure to antiepileptic drugs. *Lancet Neurol,* 2005, 4(11), 781-6.

[15]   Kluger, BM; Meador, KJ. Teratogenicity of antiepileptic medications. *Semin. Neurol.* 2008, 28(3), 328-35.

[16]   Ayhan, A; Durukan, T; Günalp, S; Gürgan, T; Önderoğlu, LS; Yaralı, H; Yüce, K. Temel Kadın Hastalıkları ve Doğum Bilgisi, Güneş Tıp Kitabevi, Ankara, 2008.

[17]   Gambol, PJ. Maternal phenylketonuria syndrome and case management implications. *J. Pediatr. Nurs.* 2007 Apr;22(2):129-38.

[18]   Hanley, WB. Finding the fertile woman with phenylketonuria. Eur J *Obstet. Gynecol. Reprod. Biol.* 2008 Apr;137(2):131-5. Epub 2008 Feb 8.

[19]   Sheard, NF. Importance of diet in maternal phenylketonuria. *Nutr. Rev,* 2000, 58(8), 236-9.

[20]   Maillot F, Cook P, Lilburn M, Lee PJ. A practical approach to maternal phenylketonuria management. *J. Inherit. Metab. Dis.* 2007 Apr;30(2):198-201.

[21]   Matalon, KM; Acosta PB, Azen C. Role of nutrition in pregnancy with phenylketonuria and birth defects. Pediatrics. 2003 Dec;112(6 Pt 2):1534-6.

[22]   Penchaszadeh, VB. Preventing Congenital Anomalies in Developing Countries. *Community Genet,* 2002, 5, 61–69.

[23]   WHO: Primary health care approaches for prevention and control of congenital and genetic disorders (WHO/HGN/WG/00.1). Geneva,WHO, 2000.

[24]   Levy, HL; Ghavami M. Maternal phenylketonuria: a metabolic teratogen. *Teratology.* 1996 Mar;53(3):176-84.

[25]   Karger, S; Führer-Sakel, D. Thyroid diseases and pregnancy. *Med. Klin. (Munich).* 2009 Jun 15;104(6):450-6.

[26]   Kyriazopoulou, V; Michalaki M, Georgopoulos N, Vagenakis AG. Recommendations for thyroxin therapy during pregnancy. *Expert Opin. Pharmacother.* 2008;9(3):421-7.

[27]   American Thyroid Association. *Thyroid Disease and Pregnancy.* 2005,

[28]   Bach-Huynh, TG; Jonklaas J. Thyroid medications during pregnancy. *Ther. Drug Monit.* 2006 Jun;28(3):431-41.

[29]   Wolfberg, AJ; Lee-Parritz, A; Peller, AJ; Lieberman, ES. Obstetric and neonatal outcomes associated with maternal hypothyroid disease. *J. Matern Fetal Neonatal. Med.* 2005 Jan;17(1):35-8.

[30]   Hong, T; Paneth N. Maternal and infant thyroid disorders and cerebral
        palsy. *Semin. Perinatol.* 2008 Dec;32(6):438-45.

[31]   The Endocrine Society. Management of thyroid dysfunction during
        pregnancy and postpartum: an Endocrine Society clinical practice
        guideline. Chevy Chase (MD): The Endocrine Society; 2007
        http://www.endo-society.org/guidelines/Current-Clinical-Practice-
        Guidelines.cfm.

[32]   Tuccori, M; Testi, A; Antonioli, L; Fornai, M; Montagnani, S; Ghisu,
        N; Colucci, R; Corona, T; Blandizzi, C; Del Tacca, M. Safety concerns
        associated with the use of serotonin reuptake inhibitors and other
        serotonergic/noradrenergic antidepressants during pregnancy: a review.
        Clin. Ther. 2009 Jun;31 Pt 1:1426-53.

[33]   Frayne, J; Nguyen, T; Allen, S; Rampono. J. Motherhood and mental
        illness: Part 1 - toward a general understanding. *Aust. Fam. Physician.*
        2009 Aug;38(8):594-600.

[34]   Yonkers, KA; Wisner, KL; Stewart, DE; Oberlander, TF; Dell, DL;
        Stotland, N; Ramin, S; Chaudron, L; Lockwood, C. The management
        of depression during pregnancy: a report from the American
        Psychiatric Association and the American College of Obstetricians and
        Gynecologists. *Obstet. Gynecol.* 2009 Sep;114(3):703-13.

[35]   Frayne, J; Nguyen, T; Allen, S; Rampono, J. Motherhood and mental
        illness--part 2--management and medications. *Aust. Fam. Physician.*
        2009 Sep;38(9):688-92.

[36]   Menon, SJ. Psychotropic medication during pregnancy and lactation.
        Arch. Gynecol. Obstet. 2008 Jan;277(1):1-13.

[37]   Einarson, A. Risks/safety of psychotropic medication use during
        pregnancy--Motherisk Update 2008. *Can. J. Clin. Pharmacol.* 2009
        Winter;16(1):e58-65. Epub 2009 Jan 22.

[38]   Use of psychoactive medication during pregnancy and possible effects
        on the fetus and newborn. Committee on Drugs. American Academy of
        Pediatrics. *Pediatrics.* 2000 Apr;105(4 Pt 1):880-7.

[39]   Davis, RL; Rubanowice, D; McPhillips, H; Raebel, MA; Andrade, SE;
        Smith, D; Yood, MU; Platt, R; HMO Research Network Center for
        Education, Research in Therapeutics. Risks of congenital
        malformations and perinatal events among infants exposed to
        antidepressant medications during pregnancy. *Pharmacoepidemiol.
        Drug Saf.* 2007 Oct;16(10):1086-94.

Chapter IV

Nutrition

Nutrition (also called nourishment or aliment) is the provision, to cells and organisms, of the materials necessary (in the form of food) to support life. The process by which living organisms obtain food and use it for growth, metabolism, and repair [1]. Nutrition includes the foods that provide energy and health, including proteins, carbohydrates, fats, vitamins, minerals and water. A nutritional deficiency is a state where an individual's intake of nutrients is insufficient for the body's normal functioning. The special physiology of a woman creates variable nutritient requirements during different stages of the life cycle [2].

Providing nutritional assessment, education, and interventions to encourage an optimal state of health may also benefit the many women who do not desire pregnancy. For these women, the provision of nutritional care as part of a periodic health assessment can be a mechanism for promoting their health over the short term, with the potential for preventing problems in the event of an unplanned pregnancy and for preventing or retarding the development of chronic diseases later in life.

The healthcare provider should pay special attention to women with regard to weight gain and nutritional counseling. The current dietary recommendations developed by the Institute of Medicine (IOM) [3] include:

a.   Increased intake of protein from 60-80 g/day
b.   300 additional calories per day
c.   Increased iron intake from 18 to 27 g/day and increased folate consumption from 400 to 600 mcg/day

Nutritional care during antepartum period should include assessment of nutritional risk factors, nutritional assessment, nutritional knowledge, and nutrient supplements, as appropriate. Some risk factors for nutritional problems include adolescence, low income, cigarette smoking, substance use or abuse, history of frequent dieting, vegan diet, pica, high parity, physical or mental illness (including depression), use of certain medications such as phentoin, mental retardation, chronic disease, and disorders, and disordered eating [2].

The nutrition-related health conditions that have been most closely linked to unfavorable pregnancy outcomes. Data are also lacking on the relationship of multiple socioeconomic problems prior to conception and the risk of nutrition-related difficulties during pregnancy. Although individually rare, birth defects taken together account for a significant proportion of mortality and morbidity among infants and children in populations where nutritional deficiencies have for the most part been corrected. Birth defects are caused by a lack of nutrients [4].

Micronutrients

Micronutrients are vitamins and minerals that are only needed in very small quantities by the body but are important for normal functioning, growth and development. In low and middle-income countries, many women have poor diets and are deficient in nutrients and micronutrients which are required for good health. Women in low-income countries often consume inadequate levels of micronutrients due to limited intake of animal products, fruits, vegetables, and fortified foods [5].

Micronutrient status may play an important role in pregnancy and birth outcomes. In pregnancy, with the need to provide nutrition for the baby too, these mothers often become even more deficient and this can impact, not only on their heath, but that of their babies too. The resulting micronutrient deficiencies are exacerbated in pregnancy, leading to potentially adverse effects on the mother such as anemia, hypertension, and complications of labor and even death [5].

Several researchers conducted systematic reviews and meta-analyses to evaluate the protective effect of folic acid-fortified multivitamin supplements on other congenital anomalies and reported that maternal consumption of folic acid-containing prenatal multivitamins was associated with decreased risk for several congenital anomalies, not only NTDs including cardiovascular anomalies, conotruncal and septal defects, orofacial clefts, limb deficiencies, urinary tract defects, nonsyndromic omphalocele imperforate anus etc. No effects were shown in preventing Down syndrome, pyloric stenosis, undescended testis, or hypospadias. These data have major public health implications, because until now fortification of only folic acid has been encouraged. This approach should be reconsidered. For the time being, women should consider the daily use of a folic acid-containing multivitamin supplement. This, along with a healthy diet, is a rational approach to preventing birth defects that is simple, inexpensive, and consistent with current data [6,7].

Poor dietary intake of vitamins has been associated with an increased risk of miscarriage, therefore supplementing women with vitamins either prior to or in early pregnancy may help prevent miscarriage [8].

Vitamin A

Vitamin A is a fat-soluble vitamin. Vitamin A is essential for normal maintenance and functioning of body tissues, and for growth and development. Vitamin A helps form and maintains healthy teeth, skeletal and soft tissue, mucous membranes, and skin. It is also known as retinol because it produces the pigments in the retina of the eye. Vitamin A promotes good vision, especially in low light. It may also be needed for reproduction and breast-feeding.

Vitamin A comes from animal sources, such as eggs, meat, milk, cheese, cream, liver, kidney, cod, and halibut fish oil. However, all of these sources -- except for skim milk that has been fortified with Vitamin A are high in saturated fat and cholesterol. Sources of beta-carotene are carrots, pumpkin, sweet potatoes, winter squashes, cantaloupe, pink grapefruit, apricots, broccoli, spinach, and most dark green, leafy vegetables. The more intense the color of a fruit or vegetable, the higher the beta-carotene content Vitamin A. These vegetable sources of beta-carotene are free of fat and cholesterol [9].

Vitamin A deficiency (VAD) affects millions of women and children worldwide. VAD is a public health problem in more than half of all countries, especially in Africa and South-East Asia, hitting hardest young children and pregnant women in low-income countries. It is common in developing countries but rarely seen in developed countries [10].

Vitamin A deficiency in pregnancy is known to result in night blindness, to increase the risk of maternal mortality and is associated with premature birth, intrauterine growth retardation, and low birthweight and abruptio placentae [11]. Vitamin A deficiency is the leading cause of preventable blindness in children and increases the risk of disease and death from severe infections. Subclinical deficiency can also be a problem, as it may increase children's risk of developing respiratory and diarrheal infections, decrease growth rate, slow bone development, and decrease likelihood of survival from serious illness. Vitamin A deficiency also diminishes the ability to fight infections [12].

A deficiency is also high among pregnant women in many developing countries. Vitamin A deficiency also contributes to maternal mortality and other poor outcomes in pregnancy and lactation. For pregnant women in high-risk areas, vitamin A deficiency occurs especially during the last trimester when demand by both the unborn child and the mother is highest. The mother's deficiency is demonstrated by the high prevalence of night blindness during this period. The impact of VAD on mother-to-child HIV transmission needs further investigation.

At least 50 million pregnant women in low-income countries are anemic, primarily due to iron deficiency. Maternal intake of vitamin A is associated with reduced risk of cleft palate decreased maternal mortality and the prevalence of iron-deficiency anaemia [5,13].

Women who received vitamin A for at least three months before and during pregnancy, weekly vitamin A supplementation reduced maternal mortality by 40% [5]. In such situations the recommended approach is to provide a vitamin A supplement during pregnancy at a dosage and frequency that will safely meet the needs of growing maternal and fetal tissue and will potentially build maternal body stores in anticipation of lactation. However, using high-dose vitamin A supplements to build maternal stores during pregnancy createds a dilemma because of the vitamin's potential teratogenicity during the early stages of pregnancy.

WHO has received requests for program guidance on the safe use of vitamin A supplements by women of reproductive age. WHO convened a consultation to consider both the safe dosage of vitamin A during pregnancy and the first six months postpartum, and the relevant policy and program implications.

Vitamin B

The vitamins B are eight water-soluble vitamins that play important roles in cell metabolism. The vitamins B are necessary in order to:

- Support and increase the rate of metabolism
- Maintain healthy skin and muscle tone
- Enhance immune and nervous system function
- Promote cell growth and division—including that of the red blood cells that help prevent anemia.

Vitamin B$_6$, also called pyridoxine, is essential in the breakdown of carbohydrates, proteins and fats. Pyridoxine is also used in the production of red blood cells. Pyridoxine can be found in many foods. Some of the foods that contain it are: liver, meat, brown rice, fish, butter, wheat germ, whole grain cereals, and soybeans. Suboptimal vitamin B6 status has been observed among pregnant and lactating women in studies [5]. Low Vit B6 levels play a role in the pathogenesis of preeclampsia [14].

Vitamin B$_{12}$ also called Cobalamin, is necessary for processing carbohydrates, proteins and fats and to help make all of the blood cells in our bodies. B$_{12}$ deficiency is a reduction in vitamin B$_{12}$ from inadequate dietary intake or impaired absorption. The condition is commonly asymptomatic, but can also present as anemia characterized by enlarged blood corpuscles with characteristic changes in neutrophils, known as megaloblastic anemia. In serious cases deficiency can potentially cause severe and irreversible damage to the nervous system, including subacute combined degeneration of spinal cord. The anemia is thought to be due to problems in DNA synthesis, specifically in the synthesis of thymine, which is dependent on products of the methylenetetrahydro (MTR) reaction. Other blood cell types such as white blood cells and platelets are often also low. Bone marrow examination may show megaloblastic hemopoiesis. The anemia responds completely to vitamin B$_{12}$; the neurological symptoms (if any) respond partly or completely, depending on prior severity and duration. Low breast milk concentrations B$_{12}$ were reported in studies [5].

Vitamin B$_9$ (Folic acid) Vitamin B$_9$ also called folic acid, (pteroy-lglutamic acid) is a water-soluble vitamin B that is involved in single-carbon transfers that are an integral part of important processes, including the synthesis of nucleotides and a variety of methylation reactions that occur in several cell compartments. The activity of the variant methylenetetrahydrofolate reductase (MTHFR) is enhanced by folate, leading to a decrease in plasma homocysteine levels. Folic asit is reguired to make DNA. The synthesis of DNA is dependent on sufficient folic asit/folate to maket the base pairs. Folates are required for purine and thymine synthesis. Without sufficient folate, cell division is slowed and urasil, rather than thymine, is incorparated into. Folic acid has two forms, dietary polyglutamate folate and synthetic monoglutamate folic acid. These two forms have different modes (active and passive) of absorption from the gastrointestinal tract, and their levels have to be combined when calculating the dose of folic acid. Estimated requirements of folate from food were also based on providing enough folate to keep most people from having folate deficiency anemia [15]. Folic acid or folic acid-containing multivitamin supplementation offers a breakthrough in the primary prevention of NTD and some other congenital anomalies [16]. Folic acid deficiency can lead to haematological consequences, pregnancy complications and congenital malformations but, again, the association with other birth outcomes is equivocal. A clinical trial by Botto et al [6] has demonstrated a protective effect of multivitamin supplements and folic acid against neural tube defects and other defects, such as orofacial clefts and some heart defects, although the evidence is not as consistent or as strong as with neural tube defects. Periconceptional folate supplementation was found to have a strong protective effect against neural tube defects [7,17].

The neural tube normally closes within 28 days after conception and other major malformations develop within 12 weeks of gestation. Therefore, folic acid supplementation should be started from 4 weeks before to 12 weeks after conception to reduce the risk of having fetuses or newborns afflicted with major malformations. If a woman has a history of a malformed offspring, she should consult her doctor on periconceptional supplementation, avoid alcohol, drugs, and smoking, consume well-balanced meals comprising vegetables, fruits and carbohydrates, and reduce the amount of lipids in food. Folate consumed in foods is in the form of polyglutamates and that present in supplements or fortified food is in the form of monoglutamates. To be metabolized in the body, the former has to be converted to the latter form. Moreover, the bioavailability of the former is relatively low, that is, 50%, whereas that of the latter is as high as 85%. Since many of the women don't fulfill the recommended dietary intake of folic acid with 400 mg/day, it is suggested that the pregnant women needed to change their dietary habits in terms of consuming more folate-rich foods and/or folate supplements [16,18].

Folic Acid Supplementation

Fortification is the first priority. Because mandatory fortification of cereal grains (e.g., wheat flours, corn flours, and rice) with folic acid (pteroylmonoglutamic acid) will maximize birth defects prevention and improve folate nutrition for the general population. Folic acid fortification of grains is safe and should result in a 20–50% reduction in rates of spina bifida, a substantial reduction in serum homocysteine concentrations and will virtually eliminate folate-deficiency anemia. Total prevention of folic acid–preventable birth defects is likely to require complementary folic acid pill programs and/or increases in the concentration of folic acid in fortified foods. Fortification with iron and vitamin B_{12} should be considered, but folic acid fortification should not be delayed because of issues raised regarding iron or vitamin B_{12} [19]. The highest-priority programs are fortification programs. Where fortification programs are not implemented or are insufficient, supplement programs can be implemented as a secondary priority and a less successful prevention strategy [20].

There are some safety concerns related to large-dose folic acid supplementation of such as masking B_{12} deficiency-induced anemia and a possible risk of increasing malignant neoplasia in the colorectum [16]. Supplementation with folic acid alone is much cheaper than multivitamin supplementation. There is no multivitamin product containing "only" folic acid or vitamins B_{12}, B_6, and B_2 currently available that could be used for the prevention of NTD and some other congenital anomalies [21].

The fortification process should include regulatory oversight of quality control in the mills and monitoring of the concentration of folic acid in fortified products. Serum/plasma folates in subgroups of the population should be measured to assess the effectiveness of fortification programs. Congenital anomalies outcomes in the population should be monitored, including spina bifida and anencephaly, folate-deficiency anemia, and mortality from heart attacks and strokes as well as the rate, severity, and course of vitamin B12 deficiency neuropathy. Products (capsules, pills, tablets, food/dietary supplements, and/or drugs) with at least 400 mcg of folic acid should be widely available and accessible without financial or other barriers. Products with 4 or 5 mg of folic acid should be widely available without financial or other barriers for women who have had a previous pregnancy affected by an NTD, and for other women who wish to have the extra level of protection from this higher dose. Currently, health agencies in many countries have officially recommended the periconceptional consumption of folic acid in the range of 400 to 500 mg/day to those young women capable of conceiving or planning to conceive [22].

The epidemic of diseases caused by folate defiency worldwide is sufficient to create a public health emergency, requiring the immediate fortification of flour and other centrally processed food staples. Public health education campaigns should be considered as one possible strategy to increase the consumption of foods rich in natural folates. To increase public awareness of the value of preconceptional folic acid-containing multivitamin supplementation, and uptake, requires a strong and widespread educational campaign to stress the importance of commencing folic acid or multivitamin supplementation immediately after the discontinuation of oral or other methods of contraception, when couples wish to have a baby. Periconceptional care, in addition to its other benefits, is the optimal time at which to introduce periconceptional folic acid-containing multivitamin supplementation, and ensures a good cost-benefit balance [17,19,21].

The primary prevention of NTD by periconceptional intake of folic acid is a major public health opportunity and has wide implications in reducing mortality and morbidity. A global folic acid technical assistance and advocacy center should be established, dedicated to increasing the pace at which folic acid–preventable spina bifida and anencephaly and other folate-deficiency diseases are prevented. This group should be charged with providing assistance to implement effective strategies that increase folic acid consumption and helping to establish systems that can track the process and outcome of folic acid programs to prevent NTDs. Such systems may include NTD surveillance as well as surveys of serum folate concentrations in women of reproductive age [7,15,17].

Iodine

Iodine is a chemical element as are oxygen, hydrogen, and iron. It occurs in a variety of chemical forms, the most important being: iodine (I-); iodate (IO3-), and elemental iodine (I2). It is present in fairly constant amounts in seawater but its distribution over land and fresh water is uneven. Deficiency is especially associated with high new mountains (e.g., Himalayas, Andes, Alps) and areas of frequent flooding, but many other areas are also deficient (e.g., Central Africa, Central Asia, much of Europe) [23].

Approximately 100 million women of reproductive age suffer from iodine deficiency [5]. Iodine deficiency can have serious consequences, causing abnormal neuronal development, mental and growth retardation, congenital abnormalities, spontaneous abortion and miscarriage, congenital hypothyroidism, and infertility. Later in life, intellectual impairment reduces employment prospects and productivity. Severe iodine deficiency in the mother can lead to impaired fetal brain development, and is probably the most important cause of mental retardation in arid or mountainous areas where iodine deficiently is prevalent. Thus iodine deficiency, as the single greatest preventable cause of mental retardation, is an important public-health problem. UNICEF has estimated that 50 million people worldwide live with cretinism and mental retardation due to iodine deficiency disorder [24]. In order to avoid adverse effects on the fetus and the consequences of cretinism and mental and growth retardation, maternal iodine deficiency must be corrected before conception.

Iodine, a volatile trace element, is more abundant in the sea than on land. Except in certain geological regions iodine has been largely depleted from world soils. Plants do not require iodine for healthy growth, and the amount of iodine in plants and animals generally reflects the low levels in soil. Thus to prevent iodine deficiency, most populations need supplementation. The accepted strategy for eliminating iodine deficiency is universal salt iodization, which is among the most cost-effective health interventions.

The current global campaign to prevent iodine deficiency by universal salt iodization is likely to lead to a significant reduction in such mental handicap. Many developing countries have been implementing this strategy, and access to iodized salt in iodine-deficient areas has increased significantly over the past decade [24,25]. Several international groups have made recommendations, which are fairly similar. ICCIDD, WHO, and UNICEF recommend the following daily amounts: age 0-7 years, 90 micrograms (mcg); age 7-12 years, 120 mcg; older than 12 years, 150 mcg; and pregnant and lactating women, 200 mcg.

Iron

Iron is essential to nearly all known organisms. In cells, iron is generally stored in the centre of metalloproteins, because "free" iron (which binds non-specifically to many cellular components) can catalyses production of toxic free radicals. Iron deficiency can lead to iron deficiency anemia. [26]. Iron functions primarily as a carrier of oxygen in the blood.

Good sources of dietary iron include red meat, fish, poultry, lentils, beans, leaf vegetables, tofu, chickpeas, black-eyed peas, fortified bread, and fortified breakfast cereals. Iron in low amounts is found in molasses, teff and farina [27]. Iron sources for vegetarians include iron-fortified breakfast cereals, spinach, kidney beans, black-eyed peas, lentils, turnip greens, molasses, whole wheat breads, peas, and some dried fruits (dried apricots, prunes, raisins) [28].

Iron deficiency results in anaemia, which may increase the risk of death from haemorrhage after delivery although its effects on fetal development and birth outcomes are still unclear.

At least 50 million pregnant women in low-income countries are anaemic, primarily due to iron deficiency [5]. Pregnant women are at special risk of low iron levels and are often advised to supplement their iron intake.

Zinc

Zinc is an essential trace element for humans, animals and plants. It is vital for many biological functions and plays a crucial role in more than 300 enzymes in the human body. The adult body contains about 2-3 grams of zinc. Zinc is found in all parts of the body: it is in organs, tissues, bones, fluids and cells. Muscles and bones contain most of the body's zinc (90%). Zinc is necessary for many biochemical reactions and also helps the immune system function properly. Particularly high concentrations of zinc are in the prostate gland and semen. Zinc plays a vital role in fertility. Zinc is especially important during pregnancy, for the growing fetus whose cells are rapidly dividing. Zinc also helps to avoid congenital abnormalities and pre-term delivery. Zinc is vital in activating growth - height, weight and bone development - in infants, children and teenagers. In females, zinc can help treat menstrual problems and alleviate symptoms associated with premenstrual syndrome [29].

Among all the vitamins and minerals, zinc shows the strongest effect on our all-important immune system. Zinc plays a unique role in the T-cells. Low zinc levels lead to reduced and weakened T-cells which are not able to recognize and fight off certain infections.

Pregnant women and lactating mothers often require more zinc. The major sources of zinc are (red) meat, poultry, fish and seafood, and dairy products. Zinc is also found in beans, nuts, almonds, whole grains, pumpkin seeds, sunflower seeds and blackcurrant. Soil conservation is needed to make sure that crop rotation will not deplete the zinc in soil. Zinc is most available to the body from meat. The bioavailability of plant-based foods is generally lower due to dietary fibre and phytic acid which inhibit the absorption of zinc. Sources of zinc for vegetarians include many types of beans (white beans, kidney beans, and chickpeas), zinc-fortified breakfast cereals, wheat germ, and pumpkin seeds. Milk products are a zinc source for lacto vegetarians [29,30].

Pregnant women and lactating mothers require more zinc to ensure optimal development of the fetus and newborn baby.

Zinc deficiency affects the most vulnerable segments of a population – pregnant women and young children, especially in developing countries. Anestimated 82% of pregnant women worldwide have inadequate intakes of zinc to meet the normative needs of pregnancy [5].

Zinc deficiency has been associated with complications of pregnancy and delivery such as preeclampsia and premature rupture of membranes as well as with growth retardation, congenital abnormalities and retarded neuro behavioral and immunological development in the fetus [5].

A balanced diet is the best way to provide your body with zinc. A zinc supplement or a daily multi-vitamin/multi-mineral supplement may be taken if her nutritional intake is insufficient. Recommended daily intakes are 15 mg for pregnant women and 16 mg for lactating women [29,30].

Multi-Micronutrients

There is strong evidence primarily that zinc, iron, calcium , magnesium and multivitamin supplementation use during the first and second trimester of pregnancy could improve birthweight, prematurity, preterm delivery and anaemia and hypertension particularly in high-risk groups. Improving maternal iron intake during pregnancy has been shown to improve the iron status of newborns. When multiple supplements were provided to HIV positive pregnant women, the risk of low birth weight decreased by 44% and by 39% for preterm births. Daily supplements of vitamin A (retinol) with iron (elemental iron) increased haemoglobin and had a greater impact on reducing anaemia in pregnant women than iron alone. While absorption of both zinc and iron are inhibited when combined, improvements in both iron and zinc status were found among pregnant women receiving supplements. The risk of low birth weight was reduced approximately twofold with multivitamin supplement use during the first and second trimester of pregnancy although it appeared that this effect was due to an associated two-fold reduction in the risk of preterm delivery [5].

Deficiencies of other minerals such as magnesium, selenium, copper, and calcium have also been associated with complications of pregnancy, childbirth or fetal development. Magnesium deficiency especially has been linked with preeclampsia and preterm delivery [5].

Another issue is that of multiple micronutrient deficiencies. The other micronutrients, especially population groups where micronutrient requirements are relatively high, in other words pregnant women and young children. This is an area of work which WHO and UNICEF are currently collaborating on which will test a multiple micronutrient mixture for pregnant women in 11 countries [29].

In a systematic review of Cochrane Database, nine trials undertaken in low or middle-income countries involving 15,378 women, a reduction was found in low birthweight and small-for-gestational-age babies and anaemia in mothers but these effects were lost when multi-micronutrient supplements were compared with iron folic acid supplements [6].

Vegetarian Diet

A vegetarian diet focuses on plants for food. These include fruits, vegetables, dried beans and peas, grains, seeds and nuts. There is no single type of vegetarian diet. Instead, vegetarian eating patterns usually fall into the following groups:

- The vegan diet, which excludes all meat and animal products
- The lacto vegetarian diet, which includes plant foods plus dairy products
- The lacto-ovo vegetarian diet, which includes both dairy products and eggs [31].

Nutrients that vegetarians may need to focus on include protein, iron, calcium, zinc, and vitamin B_{12}.

Several studies found a strongly increased risk of hypospadias associated with a maternal diet lacking in fish and meat. Mothers with a vegetarian diet in the first half of pregnancy have a five times greater risk of having a boy with hypospadias, a birth defect of the penis, compared with mothers who include meat in their diets. There is biological evidence that vegetarians have a greater exposure to phytoestrogens and thus a causal link is biologically feasible. It has been suggested that the risk of genital anomalies in male offspring may be increased by intake of different soy proteins frequently ingested by vegetarians. Soybeans contain phytoestrogens that may produce estrogenic as well as antiestrogenic effects via the estrogen receptor. Phytoestrogens from soybeans, for instance, disrupt the masculinization of the male through interference with the pituitary–gonadal axis. Alternatively, however, the exclusion of animal proteins could increase the risk of a transient deficiency of some nutrient essential during organogenesis or placentation [32,33].

Maternal Obesity

Obesity is a global health problem that is increasing in prevalence. The World Health Organization characterizes obesity as a pandemic issue, with a higher prevalence in females than males. Thus, many pregnant patients are seen with high body mass index (BMI). The definition of obese is BMI of $\geq 30 \text{kg/m}^2$. Obesity during pregnancy is considered a high-risk state because it is associated with many complications. Compared with normal-weight patients, obese patients have a higher prevalence of infertility. Once they conceive, they have higher rate of early miscarriage and congenital anomalies, including neural tube defects. Besides the coexistence of preexisting diabetes mellitus and chronic hypertension, obese women are more likely to have pregnancy-induced hypertension, gestational diabetes, thromboembolism, macrosomia, and spontaneous intrauterine demises in the latter half of pregnancy. Obese women also require instrument or Cesarean section delivery more often than average-weight women. Following Cesarean section delivery, obese women have a higher incidence of wound infection and disruption. Irrespective of the delivery mode, children born to obese mothers have a higher incidence of macrosomia and associated shoulder dystocia, which can be highly unpredictable. In addition to being large at birth, children born to obese mothers are also more susceptible to obesity in adolescence and adulthood [34].

Evidence suggests an association between maternal obesity and some congenital anomalies. In a systematic review and meta-analysis, maternal obesity was found to be associated with an increased risk of a range of structural anomalies, although the absolute increase is likely to be small. Compared with mothers of recommended BMI, obese mothers were at increased risk of pregnancies affected by neural tube defects, spina bifida, cardiovascular anomalies, septal anomalies, cleft palate, cleft lip and palate, anorectal atresia, hydrocephaly and limb reduction anomalies. Elevated body mass index has been reported as a potential risk factor for congenital renal anomalies [35,36,37,38].

Table 1. Micronutrients Deficiency and Problems

Micronutrients deficiency	Problems
Vitamin A	premature birth, intrauterine growth retardation, low birthweight, abruptio placentae, blindness, risk of disease and death from severe infections
Vitamin B (B_6,B_{12},B_9-Folic acid)	haematological consequences, pregnancy complications and congenital malformations, neural tube defects, orofacial clefts, heart defects
Iodine	abnormal neuronal development, mental and growth retardation, congenital abnormalities, spontaneous abortion and miscarriage, congenital hypothyroidism, and infertility
Iron	anaemia, haemorrhage
Zinc	pre-eclampsia, premature rupture of membranes, growth retardation, congenital abnormalities, retarded neuro behavioral and immunological development in the fetus
Other minerals (magnesium, selenium, copper, calcium etc.)	complications of pregnancy, pre-eclampsia and preterm delivery
The vegan diet	hypospadias, a birth defect of the penis

Prevention is the best way to prevent obesity problem. As pregnancy is the worst time to lose weight, women with a high BMI should be encouraged to lose weight prior to conceiving. During preconception counseling, they should be educated about the complications associated with a high BMI. Obese women should also be screened for hypertension and diabetes mellitus. In early pregnancy, besides being watchful about the higher association of miscarriage, obese women should be screened with ultrasound for congenital anomalies around 18 to 22 weeks. The ultrasound should be repeated close to term to check on the estimated fetal weight to rule out macrosomia. Obese pregnant women are screened for gestational diabetes around 24 to 28 weeks. During the second half of pregnancy, one needs to closely watch for signs and symptoms of pregnancy-induced hypertension. Once in labor, an early anesthesia consultation is highly recommended irrespective of delivery mode. Peripartum, special attention is given to avoid thromboembolism by using compression stockings and early ambulation [34].

Healthcare providers should be evaluated need for nutritional counseling, and obtain information on eating habits, cooking practices, food regularly eaten, income limitations, need for food supplements, pica and other abnormal food habits. And also they should be noted initial weight to establish baseline for weight gain throughout pregnancy [39].

References

[1] Nuritional Deficiency. Available from: http://www.faqs.org/ nutrition/Met-Obe/Nutritional-Deficiency.html#ixzz0bYXB8uZq

[2] Simpson, KR; Creehan, PA. AWHONN's Perinatal Nursing: Co-Published with AWHONN (Simpson, Awhonn's Perinatal Nursing), 2008.

[3] Institute of Medicine. 1992. Nutrition During Pregnancy and Lactation: An Implementation Guide. Report of the Subcommittee for a Clinical Applications Guide, Committee on Nutritional Status During Pregnancy and Lactation, Food and Nutrition Board. National Academy Press, Washington, D.C.

[4] PreConception Health - A Resource to Support Preconception Health Wisdom.

[5] Haider, BA; Bhutta ZA. Multiple-micronutrient supplementation for women during pregnancy. Cochrane Database of Systematic Reviews 2006, Issue 4. Art. No.: CD004905. DOI: 10.1002/14651858. CD004905.pub2.

[6] Botto, LD; Erickson, JD; Mulinare, J; Lynberg, MC; Liu, Y. Maternal fever, multivitamin use, and selected birth defects: evidence of interaction? *Epidemiology*. 2002, 13, 485-488.

[7] Goh, YI; Bollano, E; Einarson, TR; Koren, G. Prenatal multivitamin supplementation and rates of congenital anomalies: a meta-analysis. *J. Obstet. Gynaecol. Can.* 2006 Aug;28(8):680-89.

[8] Rumbold, A; Middleton, P; Crowther, CA. Vitamin supplementation for preventing miscarriage. Cochrane Database of Systematic Reviews 2005, Issue 2. Art. No.: CD004073. DOI: 10.1002/14651858.CD 004073.pub2

[9]   Mason, JB. Vitamins, trace minerals, and other micronutrients. In: Goldman L, Ausiello D, eds. Cecil Medicine. 23rd ed. Philadelphia, Pa: Saunders Elsevier; 2007: chap 237

[10]   WHO. Vitamin A deficiency.

[11]   Ladipo, OA. Nutrition in pregnancy: mineral and vitamin supplements. *American Journal of Clinical Nutrition.* 2000;72(1):S280–S290.

[12]   The United Nations Special Session on Children in 2002 set the elimination of vitamin A deficiency by 2010.

[13]   WHO. Global prevalence of vitamin A deficiency in populations at risk 1995–2005. WHO Global Database on Vitamin A Deficiency. Geneva, WHO, 2009.

[14]   Kale, A; Kale, E; Akdeniz, N; Erdemoğlu, M; Yalınkaya, A; Yayla, M. Investigation of Folic asit, vitamin B12, vitamin B6 and homocysteine levels in preeclamptic pregnancies, *Perinatoloji Dergisi.* 2006; 14(1): 31 – 36

[15]   Oakley, GP Jr. Global prevention of all folic acid preventable spina bifida and anencephaly by 2010, *Community Genet.* 2002, 5, 70-77.

[16]   Kondo, A; Kamihira, O; Ozawa, H. Neural tube defects: Prevalence, etiology and prevention. *International Journal of Urology.* 2009, 16, 49–57.

[17]   Peña-Rosas JP, Viteri FE. Effects of routine oral iron supplementation with or without folic acid for women during pregnancy. Cochrane Database of Systematic Reviews 2006, Issue 3. Art. No.: CD004736. DOI:10.1002/14651858.CD004736.pub2).

[18]   ACOG- American College of Obstetricians and Gynecologists Practice Bulletin. Clinical management guidelines for obstetrician-gynecologists. Neural Tube Deffects. Number 44, July 2003. (Replaces Committee Opinion Number 252, March 2001). *Obstet.Gynecol.* 2003, 102, 203.

[19]   Oakley, GP Jr; Bell, KN; Weber, MB. Recommendations for accelerating global action to prevent folic acid-preventable birth defects and other folate-deficiency diseases: meeting of experts on preventing folic acid-preventable neural tube defects. *Birth Defects Res. A Clin. Mol. Teratol.* 2004, 70(11), 835-7.

[20]   Bell, KN; Oakley, GP. Update on Prevention of Folic Acid-Preventable Spina Bifida and Anencephaly, *Birth Defects Research.* (Part A), 2009, 85, 102-107.

[21]   Czeizel, AE. Periconceptional folic acid and multivitamin supplementation for the prevention of neural tube defects and other congenital abnormalities. *Birth Defects Res. A Clin. Mol. Teratol.* 2009, 85(4), 260-8.

[22]   Cornel, MC; Erickson, JD. Comparison of national policies on periconceptional use of folic acid to prevent spina bifida and anencephaly (SBA). *Teratology.* 1997, 55, 134-7.

[23]   International Council for the Control of Iodine Deficiency Disorders. Iodine Nutrition. 2009.

[24]   Penchaszadeh, VB. Preventing Congenital Anomalies in Developing Countries. *Community Genet.* 2002, 5, 61–69.

[25]   WHO. Primary health care approaches for prevention and control of congenital and genetic disorders (WHO/HGN/WG/00.1). Geneva,WHO, 2000.

[26]   Kumar, Vinay; Abbas, Abul K; Fausto, Nelson (2005). "Anemia". Robbins and Cotran: Pathologic Basis of Disease, 7th edition. Elsevier Saunders.

[27]   http://www.food.gov.uk/

[28]   United States Department of Agriculture. Vegetarian Diets.

[29]   Benoist, B. Statement on Zinc and Human Health. Department of Nutrition for Health and Development, World Health Organization (WHO) at the Conference on Zinc and Human Health, Stockholm, 14th June 2000.

[30]   International Zinc Assosiation. http://www.zinc.org/zinc_health.html

[31]   National Library of Medicine Health Topics. Vegetarian Diet.

[32]   Akre, O; Boyd, HA; Ahlgren, M; Wilbrand, K; Westergaard, T; Hjalgrim, H; Nordenskjöld, A; Ekbom, A; Melbye, M. Maternal and gestational risk factors for hypospadias. *Environ. Health Perspect.* 2008, 116(8), 1071-6.

[33]   North, K; Golding, J. A maternal vegetarian diet in pregnancy is associated with hypospadias. The ALSPAC Study Team. Avon Longitudinal Study of Pregnancy and Childhood. *BJU Int.* 2000, 85(1), 107-13.

[34]   Satpathy, HK; Fleming, A; Frey, D; Barsoom, M; Satpathy, C; Fossen, K. Maternal Obesity and Pregnancy. *Postgrad. Med.* 2008, 120(3), E01-9.

[35]   Castro, LC; Avina, RL. Maternal obesity and pregnancy outcomes. *Curr. Opin. Obstet. Gynecol.* 2002; 14, 601.

[36]   Slickers, JE; Olshan, AF; Siega-Riz, AM; Honein, MA; Arthur S.
       Maternal Body Mass Index and Lifestyle Exposures and the Risk of
       Bilateral Renal Agenesis or Hypoplasia The National Birth Defects
       Prevention Study, *American Journal of Epidemiology.* 2008, 168(11),
       1259-1267.
[37]   Stothard, KJ; Tennant, PW; Bell, R; Rankin, J. Maternal overweight
       and obesity and the risk of congenital anomalies: a systematic review
       and meta-analysis. *JAMA.* 2009, 11, 301(6), 636-50.
[38]   Watkins, ML; Rasmussen, SA; Honein, MA ; Botto LD ; Moore CA.
       Maternal obesity and risk for birth defects. *Pediatrics.* 2003, 111(5
       Part 2), 1152-8.
[39]   Davidson, MR; London, ML; Ladewig, PW. Old's Maternal Newborn
       Nursing Women's Health Across the Lifespan. Pearson-Prentice Hall.
       New Jersey. 2008.

Chapter V

Teratogens

Teratogens are agents in the fetal environment that either cause a birth defect or increase the likelihood that a birth defect will occur. Several factors make it difficult to establish the teratogenic potential of an agent; timing of exposure, different susceptibility of organ systems, indivudual variations etc. Exposure in the pre-embryonic period (0-9 days) may cause miscarriage or sometimes no defects seen as a result of fully compensation with pluripotent cells. This period is defined as phase "all or nothing". Embryonic period (the time from 15th day to 10th week after fertilization) is the most risky period for teratogenic exposures. Teratogens have tissue specific effects in this organogenesis period. For example, the most risky days for talidomide were reported as 21-36 days. Nevertheless, dose-response relationships and the genetic predisposition should also be taken into consideration. In general, exposure to teratogens in the embryonic stage assumed to increase the risk of malformation and decisions should be given according to this situation. During the fetal period (from 10 weeks to birth) differentiation and development occurs on the fetus. In this period, teratogen exposures usually don't cause major defects. Teratogens typically cause more than one defect, which distinguishes teratogenic defects from multifactorial disorders. Careful assessment of the woman's daily routine provides valuable information about potential teratogen exposure [1,2].

Teratology is the branch of medical science that studies the contribution of the environment to abnormal prenatal growth and morphological or functional development. Teratogen Information Services (TIS) unit can play a specific role in public health by providing information on the known reproductive risks of most environmental agents and conducting specific research on therapies during pregnancy. Their role has many practical results: reassuring women, reducing the rate of unnecessary pregnancy terminations, and advising on using the right drug instead of avoiding necessary therapy in both acute and chronic illnesses [3,4].

Teratogenic Agents

Maternal Infectious Agents

Maternal infections have long been recognized as risk factors for adverse pregnacy outcomes [4]. Maternal infectious agents are (virus or bacteria) that cross the plasenta and damage the embryo or fetus. Some specific infections (e.g., rubella, toxoplasmosis, cytomegalovirus) during pregnancy have been associated with adverse pregnancy outcomes, including birth defects, developmental disabilities, spontaneous pregnancy loss, and preterm birth. Rubella (before 10 weeks gestation) causes cataracts and heart defects; 10-16 weeks, hearing loss and retinopathy. Varicella causes limb hypoplasia, scarring, microcephaly, chorioretinitis. Cytomegalovirus is associated with hydrocephalus, periventricular calcification, and neurological problems. Toxoplasmosis causes hydrocephalus, microcephaly, cerebral calcification, neurological problems. The effects of most infections are unknown. An improved understanding of the effects of infections during pregnancy is important for the management and counseling of infected women. Furthermore, the identification of additional specific infections as risk factors for adverse pregnancy outcomes could lead to the development of prevention programs, such as those responsible for nearly eliminating congenital rubella syndrome [5]. (Table 1)

Immunizations

Ideally women should receive all childhood immunizations before conception to protect the fetus from any risk of congenital anomalies. If a woman comes for a preconception visit, immunizations such as Measles, Mumps and Rubella (MMR), hepatitis B, and diphteria/tetanus (every 10 year) should be discussed and given at this time if needed. Routine immunizations are not usually indicated during pregnancy. However, no evidence exists of risk from vaccinating pregnant women with inactivated virus or bacterial vaccines or toxoids. Pregnant women should be advised to avoid live virus vaccines (MMR and varicella). Rubella immunization at least 3 months/28 days (1 month) before pregnancy virtually eliminates the risk that the mother will contact this infection, which can damage the fetus severely. If a woman becomes pregnant within 28 days after immunization, fetal risk is considered unlikely. Influenza vaccine is recommended for all women in the second and third trimester during flu season (october-march) and women at high risk for pulmonary complications regardless of trimester. Anthrax, Measles, Mumps, Rubella, Yellow Fever are contraindicated vaccines in pregnancy. Polio, Plague, Typhoid are not routinely recommended except in persons at increased risk of exposure. Varicella vaccine is contraindicated but no adverse outcomes reported if given in pregnancy. Indications for vaccine that are not altered by pregnancy include cholera, Hepatitis A, Hepatitis B, Meningococcus, Pneumococcus, Rabies, Tetanus- Diphtheria [6].

Table 1. Infectious Agents and Their Effects

Infectious agents	Effects
Rubella	Microcephaly, mental retardation, cataracts, hearing loss retinopathy, heart defects, deafness, congenital heart disease; all organs may be affected
Varicella	Possible effects all organs, including skin scarring, chorioretinis, cataract, microcephaly, scarring, muscle atrophy, hypoplasia of the hand and feet, limb hypoplasia,
Cytomegalovirus	Hydrocephalus, microcephaly, encephalopathy, chorioretinitis, periventricular calcification, neurological problems, microphthalmos, brain damage, mental retardation, hearing loss
Herpes virus 2	Neurological abnormalities
Toxoplasmosis	Hydrocephaly, microcephaly, cerebral calcification, neurological problems, chorioretinitis
Syphilis	Fetal demise with hydrops, detectable abnormalities of skin, teeth, and bones

Table 2. Vaccine during Pregnancy

Vaccines that should be considered if otherwise indicated:	Vaccines contraindicated during pregnancy:
• Hepatitis B • Influenza (inactived) • Tetanus/diphtheria • Meningococcal • Rabies	• Influenza (live, attenuated) • Measles • Mumps • Rubella • Varicella

Maternal Hyperthermia

An important teratogen is maternal hyperthermia [7]. The mother's temperature may rise unavoidably during illness, and can cause neural tube defects especially anencephaly, microcephaly, microphthalmia, cleft lip and cleft palate; but it is difficult to dissociate the effects of viral or other agents producing. Several studies have suggested that hyperthermia during pregnancy is associated with an increased risk for neural tube defects, independent of infection status [8]. Antifever medications and supplements containing folic acid may decrease this risk [9,10]. Hyperthermia were observed to cause NTDs, cranial nerve palsy, facial dysmorphia, microphthalmia, congenital heart defect and clup feet. Miscarriages and mental deficiency were also related to first trimester hyperthermia [7].

Maternal Drug Use

Maternal drug use is a widely-studied risk factor for birth defects. Prescribed drugs can be studied well if there is database with pharmacy data or when they are prescribed for chronic illnesses [11].

For about 80% of therapeutic drugs, it is unknown whether they are definitely safe or definitely unsafe. Ideally, no medication should be used during pregnancy [1]. In deciding whether to describe a drug, the physician must often balance the woman's need for the drug's therapeutic effects against the fetal need to avoid exposure to it. The best advice is for the women to eliminate use of non therapeutic drugs and substances such as alcohol. If she takes therapeutic drugs, the physician may be able to prescribe an alternative drug with a lower risk to the fetus or may eliminate nonessential therapeutic drugs such as acne medication. The pregnant woman who abuses drug presents a complicated picture because maintenance of her drug habit usually takes priority over health needs. She often has late or no prenatal care, increasing the likelihood that fetal damage occurred long before she encountered health care professional [7].

The food and drug administration (FDA) has classified drugs into five categories based on their risk [12]. (Table 3)

Table 3. The food and drug administration (FDA) drug categories based on risks

Categories	Drug
Category A These drugs have been tasted and found safe during pregnancy	Folic acit, vitamin B6, and thyroid
Category B These drugs have been used frequently during pregnancy and do not appear to cause major birth defects or other fetal problems	Antibiotics, aspartame, acetaminophen, famotidine, prednisone, insulin, and ibuprofen
Category C These drugs are more likely to cause problems and safety studies have not been completed	Amino glycosides Prochlorperazine, fluconazole, ciprofloxacin, and some antidepressants
Category D These drugs have clear health risk for the fetus	Alcohol, lithium, phenytoin, phenobarbital, Valproic asit, Varfarin, tetracycline, all chemotherapeutic agents used to treat cancer
Category X These drugs have been shown to cause birth defects and should never be taken during pregnancy	Accutane, androgens, coumadin, radiation therapy, streptomycin, thalidomide, diethystilbestrol, and organic mercury from contamined food

Thalidomide causes phocomelia and other limb defects, cardiac defects, gut atresia, renal agenesis. *Diethylstilboestrol* cause to clear cell adenocarsinom of vagina or cervix, vaginal adenosis, abnormalies of cervix and uterus, abnormalities of the testes, micropenis, hypospadias, cryptorchidism, possible infertility in females and males. *Warfarin* causes hypoplastic nose and bone dysplasia like Conradi disease, choanal atresia, microcephaly, and hydrocephaly. *Valproic acid* cause spina bifida, midface hypoplasia, long philtrum, small mouth and cardiac defects. *Retinoid* (Vit A and derivations) lacking and excessive amounts both lead to the teratogen effects. Retinoid embryomyopathy is characterized by disorders such as cranio-facial anomalies, cardiac defects, central nervous system development defects and thymus development defects. Varfarin and other cumarine derivatives lead to embryopathy of Varfarin. These malformations are nasal hypoplasy, Punktat akondraplasy, hear defects, and skeleton anomalies [1]. *Misoprostol* is known to cause facial nerve paralysis, with or without limb defects, probably due to vascular disruption of the subclavian artery and an ischemia in the embryonic brain stem [13].

A variety of drugs are known to interfere with folate metabolism or prevent the absorption of folic acid. These drugs comprise sulfamethoxazole-trimethoprim (anti-microbials), methotrexate (anticancerous agent), aspirin (anti-coagulant agent), sulfadoxine-pyrimethamine (anti-malaria agent), sulfasalazine (anti-ulcerative colitis agent), azathioprine (immunosuppressant agent), antacids, rifampicin (anti-tuberculosis agent), anti-epileptic drugs, and so forth. These agents should be avoided or prescribed with caution particularly to women of childbearing age. A high dietary intake of preformed vitamin A appeared to be teratogenic and it should be avoided.

Drugs are often metabolized and excreted in urine, including drugs in the fetal system. Fetal blood levels of drug often remain high because the fetus swallows amniotic fluid that contains excreted drug products, even after the drug is eliminated by the mother.

Illicit drugs (Substance Abuse, Recreational drugs) LSD, cocaine, marijuana, amphetamines can cause prenatal damage. Illicit substance abuse increases risk for stillbirth, prematurity, low birth weight, and intrauterine growth retardation. Cocaine use causes to congenital malformations of heart, limbs, face and genitourinary tract, microcephaly, cerebral infarctions, and intrauterine growth restriction. Lithium lead to congenital heart disease, particularly Ebstain anomaly hypotroidism, goiter, hydrocephaly, NTD [1,4].

Many breastfeeding mothers are also concerned about taking medications that might affect their babies. Only a few drugs pose a clinically significant risk to breastfed babies. In general, antineoplastics, drugs of abuse, some anticonvulsants, ergot alkaloids, and radiopharmaceuticals should not be taken, and levels of amiodarone, cyclosporine, and lithium should be monitored [14].

Alcohol Consumption

The prevalence of drinking during pregnancy is also high. Alcohol use levels prior to pregnancy are the strongest predictor of alcohol use during pregnancy. Studies from different countries reported prevalence between 23 and 60% [15]. Alcohol consumption during pregnancy is significantly associated with low birthweight, cleft lip/ cleft palate, and fetal alcohol syndrome, the stillbirth and perinatal and early neonatal mortality, spontaneous preterm labor. Fetal exposure to alcohol is well known cause of congenital anomalies and mental retardasyon. Furthermore, it has recently been found that exposure to alcohol during pregnancy is associated with an increased risk of sudden infant death syndrome (SIDS) [16].

Prenatal alcohol use is a leading preventable cause of birth defects and developmental disabilities. Alcohol is a known teratogen that poses serious risk to the development of the central nervous system throughout gestation. Prenatal alcohol exposure is associated with significant maternal and fetal health risks including spontaneous abortion, prenatal and postnatal growth restriction, birth defects, and neurodevelopmental deficits including mental retardation, with fetal alcohol syndrome (FAS) being the most commonly known condition along a spectrum of effects known as fetal alcohol spectrum disorders (FASD). FAS has four criteria: Maternal drinking during pregnancy, a characteristics pattern of facial abnormalities, growth retardation, and brain damage. Alcohol use has been identified as the leading preventable cause of birth defects [4,16].

Substance Abuse

Substance abuse or chemical dependency affects all body systems and can cause cardiac, pulmonary, gastrointestinal and psychiatric complications. Illicit drug or substance use, like cocaine, heroin, and methamphetamine, is highest among women during their peak childbearing years [4].

Smoking

The prevalence of cigarette smoking during pregnancy varies between 11 and 56.9% [15]. Smoking during pregnancy can be harmful to the mother and the fetus. Regardless of pregnancy status, women who smoke are at increased risk for a wide range of cancers (i.e., lung, cervical, pancreatic, bladder, and kidney), cardiovascular disease, and pulmonary disease. Cigarette smoking during pregnancy increases the chances of premature birth, certain birth defects, and infant death. Women who smoke during pregnancy are more likely than other women to have a miscarriage and to have a baby born with a cleft lip or cleft palate--types of birth defects. Smoking during pregnancy causes placenta previa, abruption, and premature rupture of membranes, preterm delivery, fetal growth restriction, and low birthweight. Prenatal smoking can also cause sudden infant death syndrome (SIDS), and infants born to mothers who smoke are more likely to have orofacial clefts. It has been shown that smoking compromises the folate status in risk groups with an inadequate daily allowance of folate [16]

Environmental Risk Factors

Environmental risks include pollutants, chemical, and other substances to which the mother is exposed in her daily life. Noise, pollution, hazardous waste sites and consumption of tap water are an environmental exposure that has also been studied with the use of birth defect registries [11].

Ionizing Radiation

Individuals can be exposed to radiation in different ways and different situations. Exposures can occur through work, medical treatment or the use of electrical equipment at home. Types and sources of radiation vary greatly. The only type of exposure that is associated with an increased risk of birth defects is maternal exposure to x- rays. [11]. Very high doses ionizing radiation to the fetus in mid to late gestation can produce microcephaly. Nonurgent radiologic procedures may be done during the first 2 weeks after menstrual period begins. This is usually before ovulation and thus before conception is possible. The radiation dose is kept as low as possible to reduce fetal exposure [2].

Chemical Risks

Solvents

One of the main concerns regarding effects of chemicals on pregnancy outcome is exposure to organic solvents. The results of studies suggested a greater risk for spesific malformations after exposure to solvents in general: cardiac defect, gastroschisis, and especially, clept lip and/or palate [17]. The exposure to solvents should be minimized during pregnancy because of increased risk for miscarriages [17].

Pesticides

The exposure to pesticides has been associated with miscarriages, fetal death and congenital malformations, particularly clept lip and/or palate as well as central nervous system anomalies [17]. Evidence exists to support that increasingly hypospadias and undescended testis [17].

Mercury

Mercury (organic, inorganic, vapor of metal mercury) can provoke embriyo-toxic and feto-toxic effect in animals and human [17].

Lead

Lead has abortive properties at high dose in the human. The antenatal exposure to moderate concentrations can induce neurobehavioral changes. Maternal exposure should be avoided during pregnancy [17].

Anesthetic Gases

Nitrous oxide, halothane and enflurane are the most frequently used anesthetic [17].

The ideally is to prevent possible effects of exposures in the home and workplace before conception, and to bring clear, not alarming, preliminary information to women of childbearing age on the potential risks connected with work and on the precautions to be taken to avoid them. It is necessary to remind them of the measures of basic prevention, strengthened or added to necessary collective and/or individual protective measures. Pregnant women should be encouraged, for their own sake, to inform their occupational physician as soon as the pregnancy is detected. The working conditions of pregnant women and, if possible, of women who have the potential of pregnant should gradually be adapted, and employees should be withdrawn from work only if no other solution can be found. Circumstances of exposure may vary, and it is important to take in the risk evaluation process.

The measurement of the intensity of exposures by regular controls of premises and a biologic surveillance of the staff have to complement the clinical search for general symptom, such as headaches, nausea or sensations of dizziness [17].

Table 4. Teratogenic Agents and Their Effects

Agent	Effects
Alcohol	Growth restriction before and after birth, mental retardation, microcephaly, midfacial hypoplasia producing atypical facial appearance, renal and cardiac defects, various other major and minor malformation
Smoking	A baby with a cleft lip or cleft palate--types of birth defects, Placenta previa, abruption, and premature rupture of membranes, preterm delivery, fetal growth restriction, low birthweight, premature birth, infant death, miscarriage
Ionizing radiation	Microsephaly, mental retardation
Pollutant	Neural tube defect and cranio-facial and renal malformations
Hazardous Waste Sites	Nervous system anomalies, musculoskeletal anomalies, anomalies of the integument system
Solvent	cardiac defect, gastroschisis, clept lip and/or palate, miscarriages
Mercury	embriyo-toxic, feto-toxic effect
Lead	neurobehavioral changes, increase abortion rate, stillbirth
Pesticides	Miscarriages, fetal death, clept lip and/or palate, central nervous system anomalies.
Anesthetic gases	Chromosomal anomalies

References

[1]   Ayhan, A; Durukan, T; Günalp, S; Gürgan, T; Önderoğlu, LS; Yaralı, H; Yüce, K. Temel Kadın Hastalıkları ve Doğum Bilgisi, Güneş Tıp Kitabevi, Ankara, 2008.

[2]   McKinney, ES; James, SR; Murray, SS; Ashwill, JW. *Maternal Child Nursing.* Saunders; Second edition, 2005.

[3]   Clement, M; Gianantonio, ED; Ornoy AT. Teratogen information services in Europe and their contribution to the prevention of congenital anomalies. *Community Genet.* 2002, 5, 8-12.

[4]   Simpson, KR; Creehan, PA. AWHONN's Perinatal Nursing: Co-Published with AWHONN (Simpson, Awhonn's Perinatal Nursing), 2008.

[5]   Collier, SA; Rasmussen SA; Feldkamp, ML; Honein MA. Prevalence of self-reported infection during pregnancy among control mothers in the National Birth Defects Prevention Study. *Birth Defects Res. A Clin. Mol. Teratol.* 2008. [Epub ahead of print])

[6]   ACOG-American College of Obstetricians and Gynecologists. Immunization during pregnancy (Committee Opinion No.282). Washington, DC, 2003.

[7]   Murray, SS; McKinney, ES. *Foundations of Maternal Newborn Nursing.* Fourth Edition, Saunders Elsevier, USA, 2006.

[8]   Moretti, ME, Bar-Oz, B; Fried, S; Koren, G. Maternal hyperthermia and the risk for neural tube defects in offspring: systematic review and meta-analysis. *Epidemiology.* 2005, 16(2), 216-9.

[9]   Acs, N; Banhidy, F; Horvath-Puho, E; Czeizel, AE. Population-based case-control study of the common cold during pregnancy and congenital abnormalities. *Eur. J. Epidemiol.* 2006, 21, 65-75.

[10]   Botto, LD; Erickson, JD; Mulinare, J; Lynberg, MC; Liu, Y. Maternal fever, multivitamin use, and selected birth defects: evidence of interaction? *Epidemiology, 2002,* 13, 485-488.

[11]   Reefhuis, J; de Jong-van den Berg, LT; Cornel, MC. The use of birth defect registries for etiological research: a review. *Community Genet.* 2002, 5(1), 13-32.

[12]   Ricci, SS. Essentials of Maternity Newborn and Women's Health Nursing. Lippincott Williams & Wilkins, USA, 2007.

[13]   Penchaszadeh, VB. Preventing Congenital Anomalies in Developing Countries. *Community Genet.* 2002, 5, 61–69.

[14]   Moretti, ME; Lee, A; Ito, S. Which drugs are contraindicated during breastfeeding? Practice guidelines. *Can. Fam. Physician.* 2000, 46, 1753-7.

[15]   Odendaal, HJ; Steyn, DW; Elliott, A; Burd, L. Combined Effects of Cigarette Smoking and Alcohol Consumption on Perinatal Outcome. *Gynecol. Obstet. Invest.* 2009, 67, 1–8.

[16]   Floyd, RL; Jack, BW; Cefalo, R; Atrash, H; Mahoney, J; Herron, A; Husten, C; Sokol, RJ. *The clinical content of preconception care: alcohol, tobacco, and illicit drug exposures.* Mosby, Inc. doi: 10.1016/j.ajog.2008.09.018.

[17]   Robert-Gnansia, E; Saillentfait; AM. Physical and chemical factors in the home and workplace before and during pregnancy. *Community Genet.* 2002, 5, 78-85.

Chapter VI

Fertility Regulation and Preconceptional Care

Family Planning

The primary goal of family planning is to provide couples with the knowledge they need to make well-informed decisions concerning whether, when, and under what circumstances to have children. Accomplishing this goal involves education and assistance in preventing unintended pregnancies. Planning for a family of the desired size and preventing additional births can substantially reduce the number of children born with birth defects simply by reducing the total number of births. In addition, couples who have an established genetic risk of producing children with birth defects can choose whether to have any (or more) children [1]. Couples known to be at increased genetic risk on the basis of their family history, age, or results of screening test, often limit further reproduction when family planning available, and need guaranteed access to family planning services [2].

A number of experiences in developing countries attest to the importance of family planning as a basic human right of women, its positive role in reproductive health and the improvement of pregnancy outcomes. By reducing birth rate and fertility, family planning may contribute to a decline in birth prevalence of genetic congenital anomalies. It has been estimated that in many developing countries with high fertility, 2–3 children per family could reduce the birth prevalence of genetic disorders by 40–50%. Further, when combined with encouragement to complete reproduction before the age of 35, family planning can contribute to a 50% reduction of Down syndrome. Unfortunately, these programs are opposed in many countries because of entrenched traditions and the conservative influence of Catholicism and Islam. In a number of Latin American countries, for example, the all-powerful Catholic Church has consistently opposed women's access to contraceptive services. While these obstacles do not affect the wealthy, they do deny women of low socioeconomic levels access to family planning services. Healthcare providers interested in preventing birth defects should ally with the increasingly assertive women rights movements in developing countries to make family planning services available and accessible to all that request them [3,4,5].

Assisted Reproduction Techniques

As the first child conceived by in vitro fertilization (IVF) in 1978, her birth launched a field of clinical care and research that continues to grow. Currently, almost 1.0% of births in the United States are conceived through assisted reproduction with even higher rates in European countries (2% to 3%). [5]. Early concerns about the health and wellbeing of children born following IVF were allayed by a small number of studies. Some of these studies were of insufficient size to demonstrate anything other than the most catastrophic of effects; some lacked comparison data or had problematic comparators. Most of these early studies were conducted when IVF was the main form of assisted reproductive technology (ART) available and for which tubal infertility was the primary indication. The second revolution in ART came in 1992 with the first successful use of intracytoplasmic sperm injection (ICSI) in humans. ICSI has enabled a much wider range of conditions to be treated successfully, including male factor infertility and the often intractable and frustrating problem of unexplained infertility. Whilst bringing hope to millions and success to many, the introduction of ICSI, by virtue of its invasive nature and because of the type of conditions it is used to treat, raised concerns about the health and wellbeing of the children conceived [6]. Hardly any experimental knowledge about the ICSI-method was available when the method was first introduced on humans. Theoretically in the absence of natural selection of the fertilizing sperm, any structural damage inflicted by the operation procedure or even the transfer of genes that would not normally have been passed on to a child, could increase the risk of health problems in the children. The risk of birth defects is among these concerns [7].

Assisted reproduction technology (ART) includes any procedure in which both the egg and sperm are handled in the laboratory and encompasses not a single approach to conception but an array of interventions. Variations are numerous with some examples including how and when the gametes are retrieved (ovarian stimulation protocols, testicular biopsy, donor oocytes and sperm), how fertilization is accomplished [intracytoplasmic sperm injection (ICSI), assisted hatching], the timing of embryo transfer, and the use of fresh or preserved embryos. Additionally, although not included in the definition of ART, ovulation induction and/or intrauterine insemination have likewise increased. Biologic plausibility for the increase of birth defects is found in several areas of ART. Epigenetic changes, alterations of DNA function without change in the sequence, are established during 2 critical periods surrounding fertilization and implantation. Concern continues that as epigenetic changes are associated with particular cancers, the possibility of unknown complications arising in children of ART as they age is relevant. Finally, the role of infertility itself as a risk factor for birth defects and possibly imprinted disorders remains difficult to explore [5].

Although many previous series of papers and the findings from the growing cohort and other studies have been interpreted widely as being reassuring, often dismissing increased risk estimates because they were not statistically significant, the results of several recent systematic reviews and meta-analyses suggest that infants born following ART treatment are at increased risk of birth defects, compared to spontaneously conceived infants [8,9]. In a population-based, multicenter, case–control study of birth defects, ART was significantly associated with ASD secundum/NOS, VSD plus ASD, CLCP, esophageal atresia and anorectal atresia among singleton births. Compared with singleton infants, infants from multiple births were more likely to have major defects [10].

Current studies of sufficient sample size and a recent meta-analysis support a 30% to 40% increase in the rate of birth defects among children conceived through assisted reproduction [5]. For example, in a recent population-based, multicenter, case–control study of birth defects (National Birth Defects Prevention Study), ART was found to be associated with septal heart defects, cleft lip with or without cleft palate, esophageal atresia and anorectal atresia [10]. The evidence relating to the risk of birth defects is less clear [9].

Despite limitations in the design and conduct of the studies carried out to date, it is believed that the current evidence is more suggestive than not of an elevated risk of birth defects following ART. On the basis of the findings, one certainly cannot exclude the possibility that there is an elevated risk [6]. This information should be made available to couples seeking ART treatment [9].

Couples considering ICSI should be counseled about the potential risks. When specific genetic abnormalities (e.g., abnormal karyotypes, Y chromozome microdeletions, CF mutations) are identified, affected couples should receive appropriate genetic counseling before proceeding with treatment. Other genetic testing before embryo transfer (e.g. preimplantation genetic diagnosis) or during early pregnancy (e.g.amniocentesis or chorionic villous sampling) may be appropriate in selected cases [8].

Preconceptional Care

Preconception care refers to interventions that aim to identify and modify biomedical, behavioral, and social risks to a woman's health or pregnancy outcome through promotion, prevention and management [11,12].

Preconception care is the promotion of the health and well being of a woman and her partner before pregnancy [13]. The purpose of preconception care is to delivery risk screening, health promotion, and effective interventions as apart of routine health care. Preconception care could be provided in a primary, secondary and tertiary health care setting. Gynecologists, nurses, midwives, general practitioners or family physicians, internists, clinical geneticists and pediatricians have all been suggested as potentially eligible healthcare providers to deliver preconception care.

Preconception Care Work Group and the Select Panel on Preconception Care in Centers for Disease Control and Prevention announced ten recommendations to improve preconception care (8).(Table 1)

The principal goal of preconception care is to maximize the quality of fetal, newborn and infant life thought primary prevention. Other goals are to provide high risk women and risk of bearing a child with a birth defect or genetic disorder and the tests available so informed choices can be made. Preconception care is a critical, because the behaviors and exposures that occur before prenatal care is initiated may affect fetal development and subsequent maternal and perinatal outcomes [14]. The opportunity for primary prevention, to address and reduce risk factors for adverse pregnancy outcomes before conception, had led many to preconception care could be the most effective strategy to improve maternal and fetal outcome. Preconception evaluation and counseling provide an opportunity to inform women about fertility/pregnancy issues, identify some of the risks of pregnancy for the mother and fetus, educate them about these risks, and institute appropriate interventions, when possible, before conception [11,12, 13,15,16].(Table 2)

Table 1. Recommendations to improve Preconception Care

Recommendations	
Recommendation 1	*Individual responsibility across the lifespan.* Encourage each women and every couple to have a reproductive life plan
Recommendation 2	*Consumer awareness.* Increase public awareness of the importance of preconception health behaviors and use of preconception care services
Recommendation 3	*Preventive visits.* As part of primary care visits, provide risk assessment and counseling to all women of childbearing age to reduce risks related to pregnancy outcomes.
Recommendation 4	*Interventions for identified risks.* Increase the proportion of women who receive interventions as follow-up to preconception risk screening focusing on high-priority interventions.
Recommendation 5	*Interconception care.* Use the interconception period to provide intensive interventions to women who have had a prior pregnancy ending in an adverse outcome (infant death, low birth weight, or preterm birth)
Recommendation 6	*Prepregnancy check-up.* Serve up, as a component of maternity care, one prepregnancy visit for couples planning pregnancy.
Recommendation 7	*Health coverage for low-income women.* Increase coverage among low-income women to improve access to preventive women's health, preconception, and interconception care
Recommendation 8	*Public health programs and strategies.* Suggest and integrate components of preconception health into existing local public health and related programs, including emphasis on women with prior adverse outcomes.
Recommendation 9	*Research.* Advance research knowledge related to preconception health.
Recommendation 10	*Monitoring improvements.* Optimize public health surveillance and related research mechanisms to monitor preconception health.

Table 2. Goals for Preconception Health

Goals
• Improve the knowledge, attitudes, and behaviors of parents related to Preconception health
• Assure that all women of childbearing age in the worldwide - risk assessment - health promotion - intervention
• Reduce risks indicated by a previous adverse pregnancy outcome through interventions during the interconception period.
• Reduce disparities in adverse pregnancy outcomes.

The period of greatest environmental sensitivity and consequent risk for the developing embryo is between days 17 and 56 after conception. Traditionally, the first visit, which is usually a month or later after a missed menstruel period, may occur too late to affect reproductive outcomes associated with abnormal organogenesis secondary to poor lifestyle choices. In some cases, such as with unplanned pregnancies, women may delay seeking health care, denying that they are pregnant. In addition commonly used prevention practices may begin too late to avert the morbidity and mortality associated with congenital anomalies and low birthweight. Recent studies demonstrated a pooled major congenital anomaly rate woman who had received preconception care. Preconception care improved outcome of a subsequent pregnancy among women with chronic disease, particularly women with diabetes mellitus and hypertension. Screening for specific hereditary disorders, such as thalassemia, cystic fibrosis and fragile X has also been shown to reduce the number of affected newborns with these disorders. Recommendations, based on existing knowledge and evidence-based practice, were developed for improving preconception health through changes in women knowledge, clinical practice, public health programs, health care financing, and data and research activities [14,17,18].

Optimizing the health of the mother before conception is important for improving pregnancy outcome. This is particularly true for certain populations of women, such as those with medical disorders (e.g., diabetes, phenylketonuria), nutritional deficiencies (e.g, folate), and exposure to toxins or teratogens (e.g., cigarettes, alcohol, warfarin, isotretinoin), in whom preconception care has been shown to reduce neonatal morbidity and mortality [16,19,20,21].

In particular, preconception care is more important than prenatal care for prevention of congenital anomalies since as many as 30% of pregnant women begin traditional prenatal care in the second trimester (>13 weeks of gestation), which is after the period of maximal organogenesis (between 3 and 10 weeks gestation).

Preconception care should be integrated into the women's health care services. Optimized preconception care is based on a comprehensive assessment of a woman's entire medical history together with a physical examination, and an evaluation of risk factors, family history, medications, and dietary and exercise habits. An assessment of diabetes in preconception care should also focus on metabolic control and HbA_{1c}, vascular and lipid status, renal function, and should include an electrocardiogram, a fundoscopic examination and tests of thyroid function [16].

Three basic components of preconception and prenatal care have been identified; early and continuing risk assessments, health promotion, and medical and psychosocial intervention with follow-up [22].

Risk Assessment

Risk assessment directs the provider toward areas in which intervention can have a positive impact on perinatal outcomes. The healthcare providers' knowledge of perinatal risk assessments allows for anticipatory planning, individualized education, and appropriate referral [23].

Risk assessment in preconception care involves obtaining a complete health history and physical examination of a woman and her partner.

Risk assessment encompasses screening for and evaluation of risk factors through assessing the woman's history, which should include an evaluations of obstetric and medical history, infectious disease history, family history, smoking, alcohol and drug use, teratogen exposure at home or at work, medication use, and dietary habits.

Psychological aspects (i.e., stress factors, including domestic violence) and socioeconomic circumstances should also be considered during a screening consultation [11].

Preconception care should also include risk assessment of the partner, as there is increasing evidence of paternal influence on pregnancy outcomes. As men may also carry or pass on genetic risks to their offspring, it is of equal importance to evaluate the family history of both prospective parents.

Depending on screening results, risk assessment often includes routine or selected laboratory tests and/or other diagnostic examinations. Blood analysis may include hemoglobin and hematocrit, blood type and Rhesus factor, liver and kidney function tests, screening for (carriership of) phenylketonuria, sickle cell anemia and tay-sachs disease, CMV titer, herpes simplex titer, rubella titer, toxicology screen, hepatitis, HIV and other STD screening.

A search for inherit trombophlias, analyses of vitamin profiles, thyroid function, autoimmune factors, and karyotype of both partners may also be performed. Other diagnostic examinations may include a papanicolaou smear, tuberculosis skin test, urine screening for protein and sugar, and an ultrasound examination of the uterus, cervical resistance test, hysteroscopy, or hysterosalpingography if uterine disorders are suspected [23].

Table 3. Preconceptional Risk Assessment

Preconceptional Risks*	
Medical history	*Psychosocial Factors*
Cardiac Disease	Inadequate finances
Metabolic disease (Thyroid, Diabetes etc.)	Poor housing
Gastrointestinal Disorders	Unusual stress
Seizure Disorders (Epilepsy etc)	Adolescent
Malignancy	Poor nutrition
Renal disease, repeat urinary tract inf. Bacteriuria	Parental occupation
Emotional Disorders, mental retardation	Attempt or ideation of suicide
Family history of severe inherited disorders	Domestic violence
Pulmonary Disorders (Asthma etc.	*Social History*
Chronic hypertension	Race
Hematologic Disorders (Sickle cell anemia, hemoglobinopathies)	Alcohol use (amount per day)
Surgery during pregnancy	Tobacco use (amount per day)
Sexual Transmitted Disease	Marihuana, cocaine or other drug use
Viral hepatitis (or risk behavior)	Chemical use at work /home
Blood transfusions,	Exposure to radiation at work
Occupational exposure to blood	Participation in sports
Reproductive History	Age ≥35 years
History of abnormal Pap-smear	*Nutritional History*
Uterine or cervical abnormalities	Vegetarianism
2 or more first trimester miscarriages	Frequent consumption of snacks/pica
Premature delivery (14-28 weeks GA)	History of buliminia/anorekia nervosa
1 or more intrauterine death(s)	Special diet
Prior baby <2,750 g at birth	Vitamin supplement use
Prior baby admitted to neonatal ICU	Milk intolerance
Prior baby with birth defect	*Medication history*
History of infertility	Use of prescription medication
Birth defects/genetic disease	Use of over-the counter medication

(*Adapted from the AWHONN Standard and Guidelines (2003), AAP & ACOG Guidelines of Perinatal Care,2002, and Centers for Disease Control and Prevention / Preconception Care Work Group and the Select Panel on Preconception Care, 2006). [24,25]

The rate of diabetes-related congenital malformations is between 6% and 10% in all pregnancies with diabetes. Such malformations are associated with poor blood glucose control before and during pregnancy [26].

Preconceptional health promotion is increasingly recognized as an important factor influencing perinatal outcome. The addition of a prepregnancy visit and the recommended prenatal and postpartum visits has been identified as an essential step toward improving pregnancy outcomes, particularly for those planning pregnancy [27]. Preconception care in women with diabetes is essential to reduce these and improve the outcome of subsequent pregnancies. Good blood glucose control before conception and throughout pregnancy will reduce the risk of malformation, stillbirth and neonatal death [26].

After screening, couples are informed and educated on a variety of health promotion issues, including periconceptional folic acid and supplement use, avoidance of alcohol, tobacco and other drug, proper nutrition, and a plan for prenatal care. They may also be counseling on the specific risks of pregnancy based on the presence of other risk factors, which may include genetic issues or the recurrence risk of previous obstetric complications.

In recent years, more and more women who previously were told or who assumed that they could never bear a child because of a (severe) congenital anomaly, chronic disease and medication use or because they have undergone an organ transplantation are opting for pregnancy. In this respect, specific preconceptional counseling issues that are gaining importance are the impact of maternal disease on the course and outcome of pregnancy, as well as the influence of pregnancy on maternal well-being. Addressing the chances that a disease may exacerbate or that the severity may diminish during pregnancy allows couples at risk to make an informed choice whether to refrain from childbearing or opt for pregnancy.

Preconceptional Intervention

The goal of a preconceptional intervention is to modify or eliminate risk factors in order to minimize the risk of adverse outcome. The best-known example is the initiation of folic acid or multivitamin. Supplement use to reduce the first occurrence or occurrence risk of neural tube defects.

Interventions of preconception care addressed include:

- Immunization status (vaccination against rubella etc)
- Underlying medical conditions, such as cardiovascular, respiratory, genetic disorders
- Pelvic examination, use of contraceptives, and sexually transmitted infections
- Sexuality and sexual practices, such as safer-sex practices and body image issues
- Dietary modification
- Lifestyle practices, including occupation and recreational activities

- Psychosocial issues such as levels of stress, exposure to abuse and violence
- Medication and drug use, including use of tobacco, alcohol, over- the-counter and prescriptions, and illicit drugs (Smoking cessation)
- Treatment of infections (i.e. urinary tract infection, Chlamydia or other STD),
- Mental health problems
- Family history and genetic risks
- Health assessment provides a foundation from which healthcare providers can plan health promoting activities and education
- Stress to importance of taking folic acid to prevent neural tube defects
- Urge the woman to achieve optimal weight before a pregnancy
- Ensure that the woman's immunizations are up to date
- Address substance use issues, including smoking and drugs
- Identify victims of violence and assist those to get help
- Manage chronic conditions such as diabetes and asthma
- Educate the women about environmental hazards, including metal and herbs
- Offer genetic counseling to identify carriers
- Support system including family, friend, and community
- Suggest the availability of support system, if needed [16,13].

Interventions may also encompass a change of potentially teratogenic drug therapy to a safer brand for women chronic medication (i.e. anticoagulation, antihypertensive drugs) improved control of preconceptional blood glucose level in diabetic women correction of vitamin deficiencies or anemia, and treatment of eating disorders [18]. The objectives of nutritional care in the preconceptional period are to encourage women to achieve appropriate weight for height and healthful dietary habits. To this end, a periodic health visit for women of childbearing age should include assessment to identify indicators of possible nutrition problems, education relating to healthful dietary practices, and counseling, referral, or other interventions as needed to solve or reduce the adverse effects of such problems [28].

Addressing preconceptional health interventions among men, such as avoidance of substance use and certain (occupational) exposures, may also reduce the incidence of adverse outcome.

Table 4. Interventions to Improve Preconception Health

Interventions	
Diabetes	• good glysemic control • dietary counseling prior to conception
Maternal PKU	• Resume dietary restrictions prior to conception
Hypothyroidism	• Monitored and doses of levothyroxine adjusted as necessary
Oral Anticoagulant use	• Talk about the possibility of switching to a nonteratogenic agent during early pregnancy
AED use	• Seek advice from health care provider • discuss the possibility of lowering the dose
HIV/AIDS	• Screening • Treatment of HIV are recommended for women before conception
STIs	• Screening • Treating
Hepatitis B	• Consider vaccination prior to conception
Rubella	• Women who are seronegative should consider Rubella Vaccination prior to conception
Folic Acid	• Consume 400 mcg of folic acid daily
Smoking	• Encouraged to stop smoking before conception
Alcohol/ drug misuse	• Not consume
Obesity	• Counseling regarding appropriate weight loss • Nutritional intake should be provided to obese women prior to conception

(Adapted from AAP & ACOG Guidelines of Perinatal Care, 2002, and Centers for Disease Control and Prevention / Preconception Care Work Group and the Select Panel on Preconception Care, 2006).

Preconceptional care could be provided in a primary, secondary or tertiary health care setting. Preconception clinic should be run collaboratively by perinatologist, geneticist, internist, nurse-clinician and a nutritionist [18]. The preconception visits may be applied to periodic health visits for women, to family planning visits, or to visits specifically targeted to preparing for conception. An increased emphasis on preconceptional care acknowledges that achieving substantial changes in diet and lifestyle often involves making incremental changes over time. It also recognizes that the primary prevention of nutrition-related fetal malformations or spontaneous abortions is possible only if risk reduction activities begin before conception; even an early prenatal visit would ordinarily be too late for effective intervention. Addressing behavioral change before conception can allow a woman to identify constructive actions and to delay conception until she has achieved a healthier physical state—one that will increase her chances for a successful pregnancy outcome.

Healthcare provider can act as advocates and educators, creating healthy, supportive communities for women and their partners in the childbearing phases of their lives. Healthcare providers can enter into a collaborative partnership with a women and her partner, enabling them to examine their own health and its influence on the health of their future baby. The information provided by the Healthcare provider will allow the women and her partner to make and informed decision about having a baby, although the decision solely rest with the couple [13].

References

[1]   Bale, JR; Stoll, BJ; Lucas, AO. Reducing Birth Defects: Meeting the Challenge in the Developing World. Washington, DC, National Academies Press, 2003.

[2]   WHO: Primary health care approaches for prevention and control of congenital   and   genetic   disorders   (WHO/HGN/WG/00.1). Geneva,WHO, 2000.

[3]   Penchaszadeh, VB. Preventing Congenital Anomalies in Developing Countries. *Community Genet.* 2002, 5, 61–69.

[4]   WHO: Prevention and care of genetic diseases and birth defects in developing   countries   (WHO/HGN/GL/WAOPBD/99.1).   Geneva, WHO, 1999.

[5]   Wilkins-Haug, L. Assisted reproductive technology, congenital malformations, and epigenetic disease. *Clin. Obstet. Gynecol.* 2008, 51(1), 96-105.

[6]   Kurinczuk, JJ; Hansen, M; Bower, C. The risk of birth defects in children born after assisted reproductive technologies. *Curr. Opin. Obstet. Gynecol.* 2004, 16(3), 201-9.

[7]   Lie, RT; Lyngstadaas, A; Ørstavik, KH; Bakketeig, LS; Jacobsen, G; Tanbo, T. Birth defects in children conceived by ICSI compared with children conceived by other IVF-methods; a meta-analysis. *Int. J. Epidemiol.* 2005, 34(3), 696-701.

[8]   ASRM- Practice Committee of American Society for Reproductive Medicine; Practice Committee of Society for Assisted Reproductive Technology. Genetic considerations related to intracytoplasmic sperm injection (ICSI). *Fertil. Steril.* 2008, 90(5 Suppl), S182-4.

[9] Hansen, M; Bower, C; Milne, E; de Klerk, N; Kurinczuk, JJ. Assisted reproductive technologies and the risk of birth defects--a systematic review. *Hum. Reprod.* 2005, 20(2), 328-38.

[10] Reefhuis, J; Honein, MA; Schieve, LA; Correa, A; Hobbs, CA; Rasmussen, SA. National Birth Defects Prevention Study. Assisted reproductive technology and major structural birth defects in the United States. *Hum. Reprod.* 2009, 24(2), 360-6.

[11] ACOG-American College of Obstetricians and Gynecologists. Preconceptional care. ACOG Technical Bulletin 205. American College of Obstetricians and Gynecologists, Washington, DC 1995.

[12] Johnson, K; Posner, SF; Biermann, J; Cordero, JF; Atrash, HK; Parker, CS; Boulet, S; Curtis, MG. Recommendations to Improve Preconception Health and Health Care --- United States A Report of the CDC/ATSDR Preconception Care Work Group and the Select Panel on Preconception Care. *MMWR Recomm. Rep.* 2006, 55, 1.

[13] Ricci, SS. Essentials of Maternity Newborn and Women's Health Nursing. Lippincott Williams & Wilkins, USA, 2007.

[14] Barron, ML. Antenatal Care. In: Perinatal Nursing. (Eds): Simpson KR, Creehan PA. *Lippincott comp.* 2008 p, 88-117.

[15] ACOG- American College of Obstetricians and Gynecologists Committee Opinion #313: The Importance of Preconception Care in the Continuum of Women's Health Care. *Obstet. Gynecol.* 2005, 106, 665.

[16] Centers for Disease Control and Prevention. Recommendations to improve preconception health and health care--United States: a report of the CDC/ATSDR Preconception Care Work Group and the Select Panel on Preconception Care. *MMWR.* 2006;55:1-22.

[17] Korenbrot, CC; Steinberg, A; Bender, C; Newberry, S. Preconception care: a systematic review. *Matern. Child Health J.* 2002, 6, 75.

[18] Weerd, S; Steegers, EAP. The past and present practices and continuing controversies of preconception care. *Community Genetics.* 2002, 5, 50-60.

[19] Milunsky, A; Jick, H; Jick, SS; Bruell, CL; MacLaughlin, DS; Rothman, KJ; Willett, W. Multivitamin/folic acid supplementation in early pregnancy reduces the prevalence of neural tube defects. *JAMA.* 1989, 262, 2847.

[20] Platt, LD; Koch, R; Hanley, WB; Levy, HL; Matalon, R; Rouse, B; Trefz, F; de la Cruz, F; Güttler, F; Azen, C; Friedman, EG. The international study of pregnancy outcome in women with maternal

phenylketonuria: report of a 12-year study. *Am. J. Obstet. Gynecol.* 2000, 182, 326.

[21]   Ray, JG; O'Brien, TE; Chan, WS. Preconception care and the risk of congenital anomalies in the offspring of women with diabetes mellitus: a meta-analysis. *QJM.* 2001, 94, 435.

[22]   United States Department of Health and Human Services [VSDHHS]. Expert Panel on the Content of Prenatal Care, 1989.

[23]   Simpson, KR; Creehan, PA. AWHONN's Perinatal Nursing: Co-Published with AWHONN. 2008.

[24]   American Academy of Pediatrics AAP & American College of Obstetricians and Gynecologists ACOG. *Guidelines of Perinatal Care.* 2002.

[25]   Association of Women's Health Obstetric and Neonatal Nurses' Standart and Guidelines, *AWHONN.* 2003.

[26]   Ozcan, S; Sahin, NH. Reproductive Health İn Women With Diabetes – The Need For Pre-Conception Care And Education, *Diabetes Voice. 2008*, 53, (Special issue): 21-24.

[27]   Recommendations to improve preconception health and health care-United States: A report of the CDC/ATSDR preconception care work group and the select panel on preconception care. *Morbidity and Mortality Weekly Report Recommendations and Reports.* 55 (RR 06),1-12.

[28]   Institute of Medicine. 1992. Nutrition During Pregnancy and Lactation: An Implementation Guide. Report of the Subcommittee for a Clinical Applications Guide, Committee on Nutritional Status During Pregnancy and Lactation, Food&Nutrition Board. National Academy Press, Washington DC

Chapter VII

Prevention Strategies and the Roles of Healthcare Professionals

Incorporating Care for Birth Defects into Health Care Systems

Hearth care systems and the services they provide vary widely among, and even within, countries. National and local priorities, infrastructure, and financial and human resources each play a role in determining the extent and speed with which interventions addressing birth defects can be incorporated into primary care and thus made widely available [1]. Services and interventions for the prevention and care of birth defects should be part of existing health-care services, in particular those concerned with maternal and child health. They should combine the best possible patient care with a preventive strategy encompassing education, preconception care, population screening, genetic counseling, and the availability of diagnostic services. That strategy must deliver services for the prevention and care of birth defects as part of a continuum of interventions for maternal and child health. Depending on countries' health-care capacity, the services should go beyond primary health care to include obstetric, pediatric, surgical, laboratory, radiological and, if available, clinical genetic services in secondary and tertiary health care [2].

Enhancing Current Reproductive Health Services

Primary health care in almost all settings includes maternal and child health (MCH) services, which include reproductive health. The services themselves vary with the needs and resources of the community and with the level of access to secondary and tertiary care for more complex and difficult health conditions [1]. The prevention of a number of genetic disorders and birth defects will follow an improvement in the quality and accessibility of preconception, prenatal and perinatal services. The improvement of preconception care should include encouraging people to procreate in the optimal age period (20–35 years of age), public education about methods that allow couples to have children when they want them, and provision of services to make those methods accessible, rubella immunization before pregnancy, education on the avoidance of teratogens during gestation (particularly alcohol), and education on the need for and how and when to access prenatal care services. Prenatal services, including facilities for prenatal diagnosis, need to be developed to the greatest extent possible. Each mother should have the opportunity of being delivered by a trained birth attendant, in a hospital or clinic if possible. Services for newborns should aim for a situation where each neonate undergoes a complete physical examination prior to discharge to detect major and common genetic disorders and birth defects [3].

Availability of Specialists

Effective delivery of services for the prevention and care of birth defects depends on the availability of a range of specialist clinical and diagnostic services, and a primary care system that is able to use them. A nucleus of expertise in medical genetics, pediatric surgery, imaging, and fetal medicine is required, with the potential to expand to meet needs. Conventional laboratory services (hematological, microbiological, biochemical) need to be supplemented with cytogenetic and DNAbased diagnostic services. Introduction may need to be a gradual process. Over time, the new technologies will support more efficient and cost-effective service delivery [2].

Training Health Professionals in Genetics

Serious efforts need to be undertaken in the genetic education of health professionals. Undergraduate curricula for the health professions (primarily physicians, nurses, psychologists and social workers) should be modernized and the practical aspects of medical genetics included in clinical teaching. The relationships between genetics and public health should be addressed in the schools of public health. For those health professionals already in practice, continuing education programs to familiarize them with the modern concepts of clinical genetics are essential. Officials in charge of public health programs should be targeted specifically for continuing education in genetics. Although clinical geneticists and specialized laboratory personnel are scarce, efforts need to be directed towards genetics training of different health professionals, including physicians, nurses, genetic counselors, psychologists and social workers. At the same time, existing clinical geneticists should be educated in public and community health [3].

Primary Care

Primary care is provided at the local level. There are very few nurses and physicians in most developing countries and most of them practice in urban settings. The majority of people receive care at community health centers served by nonspecialized health workers or by nurses or physicians linked to specialist resources at secondary and tertiary health centers. The introduction or expansion of prevention and care for birth defects in developing countries is best undertaken in primary health care facilities. Although primary care providers may have rudimentary training and few medications or diagnostic tools, they can nonetheless provide important preventive services, such as family planning, information on the causes of birth defects, micronutrient supplements, immunization, and guidance on avoiding teratogens. By forging strong linkages with secondary, tertiary, and national health care centers and by collaborating with nongovernmental organizations (NGOs) and international agencies, primary care services can increase their ability to address birth defects within communities [1].

Secondary Care

Systematic clinical examination of newborns for congenital malformations can be a method of secondary prevention (minimization of health consequences of a medical condition) through early detection of anomalies that may warrant medical or surgical intervention. Biochemical newborn screening to detect phenylketonuria, congenital hypothyroidism and other metabolic conditions is an established method of secondary prevention of birth defects in the developed world [4]. Secondary care is provided in district or regional hospitals, which are staffed by general physicians, medical technicians, and nurses. These facilities can treat more severe and complex medical conditions and provide routine surgery; they also have access to diagnostic equipment and laboratory facilities. District hospitals can expand the services offered at primary care centers by providing essential medications and vaccinations on-site and by using mobile care teams. Medical professionals from secondary facilities can support and train community health care workers, make regular visits to primary care centers to monitor their reproductive health care, review more difficult cases, and assist in identifying patients in need of referral. Training of community health workers can include, along with the care of other conditions, instruction on the prevention of birth defects, counseling and recording of family histories, and identification of patients requiring referral [1].

Tertiary Care

Tertiary care, the most specialized health care, is provided in larger, urban hospitals. Because health care resources are limited and the operating costs of tertiary centers are high, these facilities are limited in number in developing countries. As part of reproductive care for patients referred from primary care centers, tertiary care hospitals can provide genetic screening (preconceptional, prenatal, and postnatal) and surgery to correct certain birth defects. Tertiary care centers can also serve as facilities for collecting epidemiological data, providing staff training, creating and distributing educational health materials, and conducting clinical and operational research. Support of primary and secondary health care facilities by tertiary centers can contribute to the development and maintenance of affordable, good-quality health care. Studies conducted at tertiary centers can identify common birth defects and their risk factors, also preventive strategies, and effective treatment and rehabilitation. Most important is the evidence base for determining national health priorities and community health care services. Moreover, training curricula developed at these facilities can be adapted for staff at secondary and primary care [1].

Birth Registries

Birth registries provide important epidemiological information about the birth prevalence of congenital malformations. On the other hand, they raise the awareness of health professionals about the importance of recognizing congenital malformations at birth, and have aided the institution of proper medical care [4]. Worldwide, more than 100 birth defect registries exist. Some of them cooperate closely in organizations such as the European Registry Of Congenital Anomalies (EUROCAT), which collects data from more than 30 European registries in one central database and another organization that involves many birth defect registries all over the world is the International Clearinghouse for Birth Defect Monitoring Systems (ICBDMS) [5].

Prevention of Congenital Anomalies Based on Reproductive Options

The shortcomings and difficulties of primary prevention programs of congenital malformations of unknown or complex origin have led some developing countries to follow the example of developed nations and implement mass prenatal screening programs, followed by prenatal diagnosis and amniocentesis, and the option of terminating affected pregnancies. While it is true that this strategy does not prevent anomalies before conception, it does indeed prevent the birth of children with congenital anomalies, and it is the most commonly available and practiced prevention strategy worldwide [4].

The strategies for significantly reducing the impact of birth defects has three stages. The first involves the introduction of highly effective and relatively inexpensive interventions to prevent birth defects. The second stage involves improving the care locally available for affected infants. The third involves genetic screening, in the form of (1) preconceptional detection of risk factors associated with birth defects; (2) prenatal diagnosis, with termination of pregnancy offered, where legal, as an option for fetuses with confirmed severe birth defects; and (3) neonatal screening and treatment of infants with treatable genetic and metabolic diseases [1].

Recommendations

Recommended interventions for prevention, counseling and diagnosis, treatment, and rehabilitation; [1].

Recommendation 1

Basic reproductive health care services—an essential component of primary health care in all countries—should be used to reduce the impact of birth defects by providing:

- Effective family planning,
- Education for couples on avoidable risks for birth defects,
- Effective preconceptional and prenatal care and educational campaigns to stress the importance of such care, and
- Neonatal care that permits the early detection and best care locally available for management of birth defects.

Recommendation 2

Women should be discouraged from reproducing after age 35 to minimize the risk of chromosomal birth defects such as Down syndrome.

Recommendation 3

All women of reproductive age should routinely receive 400 micrograms of synthetic folic acid per day for the reduction of neural tube defects. This is best accomplished through fortification of widely consumed staple foods. Where fortification is not feasible or is incomplete, daily supplementation programs should be provided for women before and during pregnancy.

Recommendation 4

A program of universal fortification of salt with 25–50 milligrams of iodine per kilogram of salt used for human and animal consumption should be adopted to prevent iodine deficiency disorders.

Recommendation 5

Women should be vaccinated against rubella before they reach reproductive age to prevent congenital rubella syndrome.

Recommendation 6

Education programs and public health messages should counsel women to limit or avoid alcohol consumption during pregnancy including during the early weeks.

Recommendation 7

Education programs and public health messages should educate health care providers and women of childbearing age about the importance of avoiding locally available teratogenic medications during pregnancy.

Recommendation 8

Ministries of public health, in collaboration with other government departments in developing countries, should establish regulations to reduce occupational exposure to teratogens—such as mercury and other pollutants—and create programs to raise public awareness of the health risks, including birth defects, associated with these substances.

Recommendation 9

Where possible, cost-effective interventions to prevent birth defects should be provided through public health campaigns and the primary health care system. The resources necessary for their success, including staff, training, and adequate supplies of nutrients, medicines, and vaccines should be provided as well.

Recommendation 10

Children and adults with birth defects should receive the best medical care that is available in their setting, including, where possible, medication and surgery. Treatment should be undertaken as early as possible and be provided through an organized referral process.

Recommendation 11

Parents of children with birth defects should be guided to organizations that provide rehabilitation for the child and psychosocial support for the child and family. Education policies at the national and local levels should ensure that all children, including those with birth defects, receive appropriate schooling.

Recommendation 12

Countries with comprehensive systems of basic reproductive health care that have lowered infant mortality rates to the range of 20 to 40 per 1,000 can further reduce infant mortality by establishing genetic screening programs. These programs should address severe, locally prevalent conditions with clear screening and diagnostic tests; effective, acceptable strategies for prevention or treatment; and be cost-effective. Counseling, with the goal of enabling individuals to make free and informed health care decisions, including the choice, where legal, to terminate a pregnancy in the case of a severe birth defect, should be integral to all screening and diagnostic programs.

Recommendation 13

Collection of epidemiological data on birth defects is necessary to understand the extent of the problem and identify intervention priorities. Depending on the infant mortality rate, the capacity of the health care system, and the resources available, countries should incrementally develop the following:

- National demographic data on neonatal and infant mortality and morbidity,
- Data on causes of death,
- Documentation of birth defects using standardized protocols for diagnosis, and
- Ongoing monitoring of the common birth defects in a country or region.

Recommendation 14

Each country should develop a strategy to reduce the impact of birth defects, a framework of activities by which this can be accomplished, and the commitment of health leaders to accomplish these goals.

Recommendation 15

Each country should strengthen its public health capacity for recognizing and implementing interventions that have proven effective in reducing the impact of birth defects. This includes monitoring and tuning interventions for clinical- and cost-effectiveness in the local setting.

Specific Recommendations at Different Stages of the Reproductice Cycle for the Management and Prevention of Genetic Disorders in Specific Periods of Life; [6]

Recommendations for the Preconception Period

a. Improve access and quality of reproductive health services, including family planning and encouragement for women to complete their reproduction by 35 years of age.
b. Insure adequate nutrition and vitamin supplementation (especially folic acid) to women in reproductive age.
c. Expand rubella immunization to eliminate rubella infection in pregnancy.
d. Standardize family history taking at the primary health care level for the detection of genetic risk factors and referral of high-risk patients for genetic counseling.

Recommendations During Pregnancy

a. Adequate prenatal care, nutrition and delivery services
b. Raise awareness of the need to avoid exposure to teratogens, specially alcohol, tobacco, radiation and unnecessary and unsupervised medications
c. Manage maternal conditions that can affect the health of the fetus, such as diabetes and hypertension
d. Implement programs for the detection of increased risk of neural tube defects, other congenital malformations and chromosome anomalies by maternal serum screening and fetal ultrasonography, followed by the offer of prenatal diagnosis.
e. Implement programs for the detection of increased risk of selected.
f. Single-gene disorders what are especially prevalent in the population (i.e, sickle cell disease, thalasemia), followed by the offer of genetic counseling and prenatal diagnosis.

Recommendations for Newborns, Infants and Children

a. Implement systematic physical examination of newborns to detect congenital malformations, particularly of those whose outcome can be improved by early intervention (such as congenital hip dysplasia, cleft lip and palate).

b. Metabolic screening of newborns for conditions that are clinically severe, prevalent, easy detectable at birth and derive clear benefit when treatment begins in the newborn period. The clearest example of such condition is congenital hypothyroidism.

c. Monitoring of child growth and development for the early detection of genetic disorders and intervention for secondary and tertiary prevention.

d. Psychosocial support and genetic counselling for families of children affected with congenital malformations, Down syndrome and single-gene disorders of high prevalence and severity in the community.

Recommendations for Adults

a. Promote healthy lifestyles to prevent chronic diseases, such as cancer and coronary occlusion.

b. Detect individuals at risk of developing late-onset generic diseases and offer genetic counseling and presymptomatic testing if medical intervention is feasible and beneficial.

Education Recommendations

Genetic Education of Health Professionals

a. Develop and implement educational curricula with emphasis on clinical and public health aspects of genetics at undergraduate levels for students of medicine, nursing, psychology, social work and public health.

b. Develop and implement genetic education for practicing family physicians and allied health personnel.

c. Encourage multidisciplinary educational workshop among clinical geneticist, public health professionals and patient/parents organizations.

Public Education in Health Aspects of Genetics

a. Develop and implement educational and awareness programs addressed to the general public about prevention and are of genetic diseases.

b. Encourage the formation of patient/parents organizations related to birth defects and genetic diseases.

Healthcare providers who specialize in genetics health care are necessary for leading innovation and integrating new genetics knowledge into healthcare research, education, and practice. [7]

-+

Responsibilities of Health Professionals Include; [8,9,10]

- provide counseling is before conception
- identify families at risk for genetic problems,
- guide couple through prenatal diagnosis,
- determine how the genetic problem is perceived and what information is desired before proceeding,
- support parents as they make decisions after receiving abnormal prenatal diagnostic results,
- assist families in acquiring accurate information about the specific problem,
- act as liaison between family and genetic counselor,
- assist the family in understanding and dealing with information received,
- help the family deal with the emotional impact of a birth defect,
- provide information on support groups,
- aid families in coping with this crisis,
- provide information about known genetic factors,
- assure continuity of care to the family,
- assist parents who have had a child with a birth defect to locate needed services and support,
- coordinate services of other professionals such as social workers, physical/occupational therapists, psychologists and dietitians
- help families find appropriate support groups to help them cope with the daily stresses associated with a child who has a birth defect.

References

[1]   Bale, JR; Stoll, BJ; Lucas, AO. Reducing Birth Defects: Meeting the Challenge in the Developing World. Washington, DC, National Academies Press, 2003.

[2]   World Health Organization EB126/10. Birth Defects Report by the Secretariat. 2009.

[3]   Penchaszadeh VB, Christianson AL, Giugliani R, Boulyjenkov V, Katz M. Services for the prevention and management of genetic disorders and birth defects in developing countries. *Community Genet.* 1999;2(4):196-201.

[4]   Penchaszadeh, VB. Preventing Congenital Anomalies in Developing Countries. *Community Genet,* 2002, 5, 61–69.

[5]   Reefhuis, J; de Jong-van den Berg, LT; Cornel, MC. The use of birth defect registries for etiological research: a review. *Community Genet,* 2002, 5(1), 13-32.

[6]   WHO: Prevention and care of genetic diseases and birth defects in developing countries (WHO/HGN/GL/WAOPBD/99.1). Geneva, WHO, 1999.

[7]   Lea, DH; Williams, JK; Cooksey, JA; Flanagan, PA; Forte, G; Blitzer, MG.U.S. Genetic Nurses in Advanced Practice 2006. *Journal of Nursing Scholarship,* 38:3, 213-218.

[8]   Davidson, MR; London, ML; Ladewig, PW. Old's Maternal Newborn Nursing Women's Health Across the Lifespan. Pearson-Prentice Hall. New Jersey. 2008. p: 288-291.

[9]   McKinney, ES; James, SR; Murray, SS; Ashwill, JW. *Maternal Child Nursing. Saunders; Second edition,* 2005.

[10] Murray, SS; McKinney, ES. Foundations of Maternal Newborn Nursing. Fourth Edition, *Saunders Elsevier,* USA, 2006.

Conclusion

Congenital anomalies, including genetic diseases, affect many infants and their parents and families, and if primary prevention would be possible, much suffering could be avoided. Health professionals, particularly public health officials, must be educated in the aims and methods of preventing birth defects with low cost and high impact. The basis for public health preventive measures should be the primary health care level, where identification of risks and prospective genetic counseling should be done by specially trained allied health professionals. Higher-level medical centers should be available for referral when indicated.

Index

fluid, 29, 35
folate, 40, 59, 64, 65, 66, 74, 82, 84, 94
folic acid, vii, viii, 1, 2, 6, 7, 27, 28, 39,
  41, 52, 53, 54, 60, 63, 64, 65, 66, 70,
  74, 75, 80, 82, 97, 98, 99, 101, 108,
  112
food, 59, 64, 65, 66, 70, 73, 80, 81
fruits, 60, 64, 68, 70

G

gases, 11, 86
gastroschisis, 6, 84, 86
gene, 9, 15, 24, 27, 112, 113
general practitioner, 54, 92
genetic counselling, 21, 113
genetic disease, vii, 19, 20, 96, 100, 114,
  115, 117
genetic disorders, viii, 2, 9, 56, 75, 89,
  97, 100, 104, 113, 115
genetic factors, 34, 114
genetic screening, 7, 16, 18, 106, 107,
  110
genetics, 16, 104, 105, 113, 114
gestation, vii, 27, 29, 31, 35, 37, 44, 45,
  46, 47, 49, 64, 78, 83, 84, 94, 104
gestational age, 25, 30, 46
gestational diabetes, 12, 71, 72
girls, 25, 38
glucose, 30, 38, 39, 52, 96, 97, 98
goals, 38, 92, 111
goiter, 47, 82
government, 11, 109
grains, 65, 69, 70
groups, 3, 13, 15, 16, 26, 67, 69, 70, 84,
  114
growth, 29, 35, 46, 47, 49, 51, 52, 59,
  60, 61, 62, 63, 67, 68, 69, 72, 77, 82,
  83, 113
guidance, 13, 54, 62, 105
guidelines, 50, 57, 74, 87

H

harm, 12, 41
hazards, 11, 48, 98
health, vii, viii, 2, 4, 6, 9, 10, 11, 13, 14,
  15, 16, 21, 25, 27, 37, 38, 48, 54, 55,
  56, 59, 60, 66, 67, 71, 75, 80, 81, 83,
  89, 90, 92, 93, 94, 95, 96, 97, 98, 99,
  100, 101, 102, 103, 104, 105, 106,
  107, 108, 109, 110, 111, 112, 113,
  114, 117
health care, 2, 10, 13, 14, 16, 27, 48, 54,
  56, 75, 80, 92, 94, 99, 100, 101, 102,
  103, 104, 105, 106, 108, 109, 110,
  111, 112, 114, 117
health care system, 110, 111
health problems, 4, 90, 98
hearing loss, 27, 78, 79
height, 28, 68, 98
hemoglobinopathies, 9, 96
hepatitis, 78, 95, 96
HIV, 13, 62, 69, 95, 99
HIV/AIDS, 13, 99
homocysteine, 64, 65, 74
hormone, 43, 44, 45, 46, 53
hospitals, 21, 106
housing, 10, 96
hydrocephalus, 6, 78
hydrocephaly, 72, 81, 82
hydrops, 47, 79
hyperbilirubinemia, 30, 35
hypertension, 60, 69, 71, 72, 94, 96, 112
hyperthermia, 17, 18, 22, 80, 87
hyperthyroidism, 43, 45, 46, 47, 53
hypoplasia, 50, 78, 79, 81, 86
hypospadias, 61, 71, 72, 75, 81, 85
hypothyroidism, vii, 43, 44, 45, 46, 67,
  72, 106, 113

I

ideal, 28, 49